Cancer Nur

MEDICAL

edited by

ROBERT TIFFANY SRN, RCNT
Director of Nursing
The Royal Marsden Hospital, London and Surrey

FABER AND FABER · London and Boston

First published in 1978
by Faber and Faber Limited
3 Queen Square London WC1
Printed in Great Britain by
Cox and Wyman Limited
Fakenham Norfolk
All rights reserved

© Faber and Faber Limited 1978

CONDITIONS OF SALE

This book is sold subject to the condition that it shall not, by way of trade or otherwise, be lent, re-sold, hired out or otherwise circulated without the publisher's prior consent in any form of binding or cover other than that in which it is published and without a similar condition including this condition being imposed on the subsequent purchaser

British Library Cataloguing in Publication Data

Cancer nursing.
  Vol. 1: Medical.
  1. Cancer nursing
  I. Tiffany, Robert
  610.73'6   RC266
    ISBN 0–571–11174–2
    ISBN 0–571–11175–0   Pbk.

TO MY PARENTS

Contents

Foreword by Patricia A. Downie FCSP	*page*	11
Editor's Preface		13
Acknowledgements		15
List of Contributors		17
Introduction		19

1. Cancer Chemotherapy – Principles and Practice
   by T. J. McElwain MB, BS, FRCP ... 21

2. Care of Patients Receiving Anti-Tumour Drugs
   by E. Wark SRN, FETC ... 38

3. Care of Patients Receiving Hormonal Therapy
   by G. Diggory SRN, RCNT ... 60

4. Management of Intravenous Therapy
   by M. D. Marks BA (Hons.), SRN ... 73

5. Control of Infection in a Cancer Hospital
   by E. Scott SRN, RCNT ... 113

6. Care of Patients Requiring a Pathogen Reduced Environment
   by J. Edwards SRN ... 122

7. CARE OF PATIENTS IN THE CELL SEPARATOR UNIT
   by S. D. Mackey SRN — *page* 134

8. THE NURSING MANAGEMENT OF CHILDREN WITH CANCER
   by K. Preston SRN, RSCN — 146

9. NURSING MANAGEMENT OF THE PATIENT WITH PAIN
   by P. Hinds SRN — 159

10. TERMINAL CARE
    by M. Krauss SRN, DN(Lond.) — 171

    INDEX — 187

Illustrations

PLATES

4/1	Container showing label indicating drug additive to infusion fluid	*page* 92
4/2	Extravasation from a vesicant cytotoxic agent	102
6/1	The interior of a single isolation room	126
6/2	The sterile kitchen	127
6/3	The Life Island	132
7/1	The IBM Cell Separator machine in use	137
7/2	A patient attached to Cell Separator machine while in use	137
8/1	Twelve year old patient bakes cakes	149
8/2	Mother being taught to care for the child's permanent tracheostomy	150
8/3	Three year old child receiving cranial irradiation	153

FIGURES

3/1	Hormones influencing breast tumours	61
4/1	Winged infusion devices	78
4/2	'Needle-through' cannulae	79
4/3	'Needle-through-devices'	81
4/4	A 'catheter-inside-needle' device wound on a drum	82
4/5	A bottle of intravenous fat emulsion that has 'cracked' after the addition of a drug	88
4/6	Containers which had KCl (potassium chloride) added	91
4/7	Set record labels	99
6/1	Diagrammatic representation of 16 bed reverse barrier unit	123
7/1	The theory of immunotherapy	136
7/2	The sites of injection for immunotherapy	141
7/3	The Leukopak filter	143
7/4	Cross-section of Leukopak filter	143
9/1	Diagram showing pain scale measurement	165

Foreword
by PATRICIA A. DOWNIE FCSP

A little over a hundred years ago, Florence Nightingale wrote 'do we *care* for the patient first and foremost? That is the first and last keynote. The alpha and omega is, do we *wisely look after* the patients?'

The emphasis is mine; the words are Miss Nightingale, and they sum up the ethos of nursing, and nowhere is this more necessary than in nursing of the patient with a diagnosis of a cancerous disease.

In the past decade there have been enormous developments in medical, surgical and radiotherapeutic treatments of cancer. This has placed great responsibility upon the nurse, for she is the person nearest to the patient and therefore becomes a key figure in his care. Basic nurse training ensures that the nurse is able to fulfil the prime needs of any patient – those necessary to simple comfort. The nurse who is either specialising in cancer nursing, or who only occasionally meets a patient undergoing intensive care/treatment for cancer, will need to understand why certain treatments are given, how drugs work and interact, why natural immunity is lowered, why side-effects occur and what reactions may be expected and which need to be looked for.

Any nurse (be she hospital or community based), who is involved however little, with cancer patients, will find the answers to many questions and problems in this book. Furthermore, nurses will be helped to a realisation that the diagnosis of cancer is not a certain death warrant and that with well-planned treatment excellent results can be obtained. Rightly, there is a chapter on the care of those who will die, and again the emphasis is positive and will help the nurse to accept that death is not to be seen as a failure of treatment. Throughout the book team work is stressed and the nurse can be clearly seen as a *partner* in this work with the doctors.

Robert Tiffany is well fitted to the task of editing these volumes on Cancer Nursing; he has wisely invited practical, caring nurses to outline the nursing requirements for these patients. The results are volumes of great practicality, common sense, sound technical knowledge and above all, compassion. Cancer nursing is essentially '*care* for the patient first and foremost'.

Holborn, 1977   *P.A.D.*

Editor's Preface

Cancer as a term, encompasses a multitude of diseases and is consequently frequently misunderstood. The word cancer is still considered sinister and too often synonymous with death. Oncology (the study of the tumour), is a complex subject, exciting and challenging, yet the myths associated with cancer are perpetrated even by professionals working in all Health Services. When one considers the breadth of basic training needed to prepare nurses to practise, it is understandable that their depth of knowledge in any one speciality is limited. Historically nurses are trained as generalists; yet we expect every registered nurse to know about the complexities of modern drug regimens, care for the critically ill and chronically sick patient, care for patients in all age groups and care for patients in institutions and in their homes.

As the patterns of health care change, nursing has had to adapt itself to meet these changes. The knowledge acquired by nurses during their training is extensive but it is becoming widely recognised that the need for post-basic training is essential if we are to maintain and improve our standards of patient care. Medical specialisation is a reality and it is becoming increasingly apparent that nurses must rethink their role if they are to stay in the forefront of the caring professions.

Oncology is different from other specialities in that it is diverse in the treatment modalities available and the anatomical distribution of the disease. For this reason *Cancer Nursing* has been divided into three volumes: Medical, Radiotherapy, and Surgical. Each volume takes nursing care as the primary focus of attention and each chapter has been written by nurses experienced in their field of activity. It is hoped that *Cancer Nursing* will be of value to nurses undertaking post-basic courses in oncological nursing. It is recognised however, that not all nurses caring for patients with cancer will be able to attend such courses and that the majority of cancer patients are cared for outside specialist centres in general hospitals or in the community. The contents of the book and presentation of material has been arranged with this fact in mind to enable it to be of particular value to hospital and community nurses where care of the patient with cancer constitutes only a part of their wide range of responsibilities.

Cancer is curable and many thousands of patients are a living testimony to this fact. Many thousands still die from cancer and others live with their disease under control. Nurses should show an attitude of optimism towards cancer as a curable disease, as they would to any other disease. They should recognise the value and contribution which various types of treatment make towards the cure of cancer and that where cancer is not curable, valuable palliation may be achieved. The nurse's own feelings towards the diagnosis and treatment may be projected to the patient and his family even when not expressed verbally. If the nurse cannot face up to the fact that there are diseases called cancer, from which some patients can be cured, others can live many happy and fruitful years with the disease under control, and some will die of the disease, she will be of little help to the patient and his family.

The nurse who is knowledgeable about today's sophisticated treatment modalities and who possesses the ability to show compassion and empathy will be valued by the patient, his family and other health care professionals. It is towards this goal that this book is directed.

R.T., 1977

Acknowledgements

I am grateful to the various authors who have contributed to this volume, and to the physicians who have so willingly checked the technical data.

I thank the Photographic Department of the Royal Marsden Hospital, for providing the plates and Mrs Anne Barrett for executing the line drawings.

I am indebted to Miss Sue Cox, Senior Nursing Officer, The Royal Marsden Hospital for her unfailing help and advice.

Finally, I express my thanks to Miss P. Downie, Nursing and Medical Editor of Faber and Faber for her guidance and support in the preparation of this volume.

Contributors

Miss G. DIGGORY SRN, RCNT
Nurse Teacher, Department of Nursing Studies, The Royal Marsden Hospital, London and Surrey

Miss J. EDWARDS, SRN
Sister, The Reverse Barrier Nursing Unit, The Royal Marsden Hospital, London and Surrey

Mr P. HINDS SRN
Nurse Teacher, Department of Nursing Studies, The Royal Marsden Hospital, London and Surrey

Miss M. KRAUSS SRN, DN (Lond.)
Sister in Charge, Mayneord Ward, The Royal Marsden Hospital, London and Surrey

Miss S. MACKEY SRN
Sister, Cell Separator Unit, The Royal Marsden Hospital, London and Surrey

Dr T. J. McELWAIN MB, BS, FRCP
Consultant Physician, The Royal Marsden Hospital, London and Surrey
Senior Lecturer in Medicine, Institute of Cancer Research, London and Surrey

Miss M. D. MARKS BA (Hons.), SRN
Clinical Nurse Specialist, Intravenous Therapy, Royal Marsden Hospital, London and Surrey

Miss K. PRESTON SRN, RSCN
Sister in Charge, Paediatric Unit, The Royal Marsden Hospital, London and Surrey

Miss E. SCOTT SRN, RCNT
Clinical Nurse Specialist, Infection Control, The Royal Marsden Hospital, London and Surrey

Miss E. WARK SRN, FETC
Nursing Officer, Department of Nursing Studies, The Royal Marsden Hospital, London and Surrey

Introduction

Medical Oncology is one of the most revolutionary areas of medicine today; it may truly be predicted that what is hearsay today is dogma tomorrow. Tremendous advances have been made during the past few years which have transformed the philosophy of the use of anti-tumour drugs. Less than a decade ago, such drugs were used only for palliative relief of symptoms and to treat those malignant diseases not amenable to conventional treatment by surgery and radiotherapy. Today anti-tumour drug therapy is considered as an integral part of primary therapy adjuvant to surgery and radiotherapy. New knowledge concerning the action of these drugs coupled with better systems of administration has reduced dramatically the toxic effect of these drugs.

This rapid growth in the knowledge and use of anti-tumour drugs makes it difficult to present up-to-date information in textbook form. To overcome this problem, attention has been placed on the principles guiding the use of chemotherapy and the effects of these agents both toxic and therapeutic. Particular regimens for specific tumours have been avoided because of the rapid changes that are occurring and the multiplicity of competing protocols.

In addition to the care and management of patients being treated for primary or secondary disease with anti-tumour drugs this volume also includes those measures of care and support that are vital to ensure the best possible delivery of nursing care. Care of Children with Cancer and Care of the Terminally Ill patient are included in this volume because although various modalities of treatment may be given they fall mainly within the category of medical oncology.

1. Cancer Chemotherapy – Principles and Practice

by T. J. McELWAIN MB, BS, FRCP

INTRODUCTION

The use of drugs to treat cancer is a comparatively recent development and has only been recognised as a worthwhile part of the multidisciplinary management of malignant disease in the last 25 years. The early successes of chemotherapy were with leukaemia and lymphomas and until recently there was little evidence that drugs greatly increased the quality or quantity of life of most patients with common tumours such as carcinoma of the breast, lung and gastro-intestinal tract. Here the only effective treatment was with surgery and radiotherapy which could be curative so long as the tumour remained localised and had not spread to places in the body distant from its site of origin. Although this still remains broadly true, it is now established that some patients with widely disseminated tumours such as breast cancer, oat cell carcinoma of the bronchus, testicular teratoma, soft tissue sarcoma and most tumours of childhood will benefit from drug treatment if this is properly applied. The best results have usually been obtained by specialist groups in which there is close collaboration of people from different disciplines, and where careful attention is not only given to applying the most appropriate mix of treatments but also to full investigation of the patient so that the clearest possible picture can be obtained of the extent of the disease. It is only when we know this that the most appropriate sequence of treatment can be given and there exists at least the possibility that all the tumour can be eradicated from the body.

The potential advantage of drugs over surgery and radiotherapy is that they have the capacity to seek and destroy cancer cells all over the body and not only locally. The disadvantages of the 30 or so drugs that are now available for use in man is that they are not only toxic to tumours but also to normal tissues; in other words they are relatively *unselective* in their activity. A major goal of modern cancer chemotherapy is to improve drug selectivity.

The problem of drug selectivity centres around the fact that drugs used in cancer chemotherapy interfere with the production of deoxyribonucleic acid (DNA), ribonucleic acid (RNA) and protein in the cell. Since all dividing cells, normal and malignant, require these substances, this explains the toxicity of the drugs to normal tissues. Nevertheless, an apparent selectivity for tumour tissue is quite often seen and this depends upon many different factors among which are the dosage, timing and route of drug administration, and the capacity of some normal tissues more rapidly to repair drug-induced damage than tumour cells. To understand these factors better one needs first to look at the way in which normal and malignant tissues grow and then to see how drugs can interfere with this process.

CELL KINETICS

Most tissues can renew themselves although some, such as the cells of the brain cannot. In order to divide a cell must be able to synthesise twice the normal amount of DNA in its nucleus so that its division results in two cells with the normal or 'resting'. amount of DNA. This sequence of events is known as the cell 'cycle'. It begins with division or mitosis (M) producing two cells which then spend a period of time in the first resting phase (G1). Following this there is a burst of DNA synthesis (S phase) in which the amount of DNA is doubled. A second resting phase (G2) then follows before mitosis occurs again. In any tissue, the proportion of cells which are involved in this cyclical process is known as the 'growth fraction'. Cells not involved are said to be 'out of cycle' and one of two things can happen to them. They can either remain out of cycle and eventually die, or they can remain alive and eventually begin cycling again. The rate of growth of a tissue will therefore depend upon a number of factors of which the growth fraction, the time between successive divisions of cells and the proportion of cells out of cycle and dying in the tissue are the important ones. In normal tissues cell division is a response to the need for renewal of cells that are lost from the tissue and control mechanisms exist which ensure that the number of new cells which are added to the tissue balances but does not exceed the cell losses. In tumours these control mechanisms are faulty so that uncontrolled growth occurs, and cells fail to cease dividing when a critical mass of tissue has been reached. Death follows when the number of tumour cells in the body reaches about one million million (10^{12}).

It is generally thought that cells which are in cycle are more sensitive to anti-cancer drugs than those out of cycle and this partly explains the apparent paradox that rapidly growing tumours are often more sensitive to the action of drugs than those which are slowly growing. It also goes some way to explain one cause of the failure of drug treatment – cells which are temporarily out of cycle may fail to be killed by drugs, but represent a pool from which regrowth of the tumour can occur later if they start cycling again.

These normal tissues such as bone marrow and the lining of the gastro-intestinal tract contain a high proportion of cells which are cycling. It is therefore not surprising that these tissues are frequently damaged by cytotoxic drugs and that this damage is a major limitation upon the amount of chemotherapy that can safely be given to patients with tumours. Many chemotherapists now feel that much more work needs to be done to elucidate both the way in which normal tissues are damaged by drugs and the way in which they recover from this damage with particular emphasis upon ways in which these processes may differ from those in tumours. Such differences, if present, may be exploited when optimal chemotherapy programmes are designed in the future.

An important cell kinetic concept which has influenced modern cancer chemotherapy is that of 'fractional cell kill'. It has been found in experimental animal systems that for a given dose of drug a fixed proportion of tumour cells is killed irrespective of the actual number of cells in the tumour. For example, a particular dose of a drug will kill, say, 90 per cent of the cells in a tumour. If the tumour contained one million cells that dose would kill nine hundred thousand cells. If it contained one thousand cells the same dose would kill nine hundred cells (the same proportion); it would not eradicate the tumour. In clinical terms, this is important. It means that although it may be easy to eradicate the bulk of a tumour with a drug, it is difficult to kill the small amount of tumour that remains behind unless repeated doses of the drug are given. But it also implies that the best time to eradicate a tumour with drugs is when that tumour is very small, i.e. contains a relatively small number of cells. Biologically speaking, 'small' in this context means clinically undetectable. This has led to the use of drug treatment in patients after all their detectable tumour has been removed by surgery and/or radiotherapy. For particular tumours it is known that there is a high chance that small amounts of tumour do remain in the body after local treatment and it is hoped that the early use of high dose intermittently administered drugs will eradicate these foci of disease. This is an example of 'adjuvant' chemotherapy which will be discussed in more detail later.

DRUG KINETICS

An understanding of the behaviour of normal and malignant tissues alone is not enough for the design of optimal cancer chemotherapy. One must also know about the way in which drugs are distributed in and eliminated from the body so as to achieve the maximum concentration of drug in the tumour for a time long enough for them to kill the cancer cells. Thus, the optimal administration of a drug may depend upon the route of administration, the time and duration of administration, the proliferative characteristics of the tumour, the site of the tumour and the metabolic properties of both the normal and malignant tissues. If more than one drug is given it is also necessary to know about interactions between the drugs which may be beneficial or harmful. These considerations may make drug administration very complex and are the subject of a great deal of investigation at present.

GETTING A NEW DRUG FROM THE LABORATORY TO THE CLINIC

Most anti-tumour agents have been found by chance, some have been the result of rational design based upon known properties of tumour and normal cells. Others are analogues (chemical variants) of compounds already in clinical use. The initial testing of a potential new anti-cancer agent is done in genetically identical animals bearing tumours which can be transplanted from one to another. The animal tumours in use today are those which in the past have shown sensitivity to the agents that are currently used in the clinic. It is important to stress that these are animal tumours and not human ones and that they differ in many respects from the common human cancers. The main differences are that they grow rapidly, are chosen for their sensitivity to drugs and are sometimes curable with drugs. There can be little doubt that using this system many drugs which might have been useful in man have been missed. A potentially important recent advance has been the development of laboratory mice which will accept transplants of human tumours (xenografts). The tumours will grow in the animals and retain some, but not all, of their human characteristics. New drugs are now being tested for activity against human tumour xenografts but it remains to be seen whether their use will result in the discovery of better drugs than the ones that we are already using.

If a drug shows significant anti-tumour activity in animals it must then be screened for unwanted toxicity in small (rodents) and large animals (usually dogs or monkeys). If it passes the toxicity screen it can then be licensed for limited clinical studies in selected patients with cancer. The first of these, the 'phase one' study is done to establish its toxicity – anti-tumour activity is not required – and to determine its clinical pharmacology, dosage, timing and route of administration.

Patients used in such studies must be informed volunteers in whom all available orthodox treatment has been used and failed. This can then be followed by 'phase two' studies in which groups of patients with tumours are given the drug in order to determine the extent to which the tumour responds to the drug and the effect, if any, that the treatment has upon the survival of the patients. At this stage the patients usually have very advanced cancers which have already been subjected to many other treatments, and the results obtained may not give a true indication of the effect that the drug would produce if it were given earlier in the course of the disease. If the drug shows promise it can then be used alone and in combination with other drugs in clinical trials in which its efficacy is compared with that of drugs whose effectiveness is already established. Later studies determine the way in which drug treatment can most effectively be integrated into an overall treatment programme for a particular tumour. Here, drug treatments that have been found effective in the management of advanced tumours may be used as primary treatment or as adjuvants to surgery and radiotherapy, the exact pattern of use depending upon the clinical patterns of disease that each tumour produces.

THE CLINICAL USE OF CYTOTOXIC DRUGS

Continuous, single-agent, low dose chemotherapy

In the early days of cancer chemotherapy this was the usual way of using drugs. The principle was to give drugs one at a time, and usually in low doses; and therapy was often discontinued if the tumour responded to the treatment. When relapse occurred a second drug was tried, and the process was repeated until all the available agents had been used. This type of treatment generally produced low response rates; complete remissions were infrequent and any remission at all was often short though a few patients with acute leukaemia, a lymphoma or an ovarian tumour would occasionally achieve a long-lasting remission. This type of treatment is inherently unsatisfactory; low doses can be expected to kill relatively small fractions of tumour cells; they potentiate the development of drug resistance, and they fail to exploit kinetic differences between the tumour and normal rapidly dividing tissues such as the bone marrow and gastro-intestinal epithelium.

This type of chemotherapy is now little used in modern cancer management though one should be careful before abandoning it completely. It has proved of value in the management of the chronic leukaemias in adults and some nodular lymphomas, and it might still be useful in treatment programmes for other tumours in which more intensive chemotherapy is first deployed to destroy rapidly proliferating tumour cells; low dose continuous treatment might then be used to eradicate some of the more slowly proliferating residual cells.

Cyclical chemotherapy

The principle here is to give cytotoxic drugs in a cyclical fashion, deliberately changing from one effective drug to another at fixed intervals. The aim is to prevent the tumour from becoming resistant to each drug or combination of drugs by its deliberate withdrawal before tumour resistance has had time to develop and before characteristic side-effects of the drugs become apparent. The principle is embodied in many modern treatment programmes and there is evidence that it prolongs remission.

Intermittent, high dose chemotherapy

This type of treatment forms the basis of most modern chemotherapeutic regimes. Drugs are given in high doses over short periods, separated by intervals for host recovery between courses. The aim of such treatment is to kill a large fraction of tumour cells with each course of the drug at the cost of transient reversible toxicity to the host. This is an application of the fractional cell kill principle and although there is no way of being sure that this holds good for human tumours there is evidence, mostly from sensitive tumours like acute leukaemia in childhood, that high dose chemotherapy not only increases the rate and magnitude of the response of the tumours to cytotoxic drugs but also prolongs the duration of remission that is achieved. It is less certain that giving very high doses of drugs to patients whose tumours are unresponsive to conventional doses of these agents makes much difference. Such evidence as is available is conflicting and certainly it would be folly to attempt this type of treatment except under controlled conditions in special centres where there is a high level of chemotherapeutic expertise; it must be remembered that despite manoeuvres designed to exploit kinetic differences between neoplastic and normal cells, the margin between increased tumour eradication and toxicity to the host is narrow. Cancer chemotherapy can be a form of clinical tightrope walking: used injudiciously, high dose chemotherapy can result in severe and at times irreversible toxicity to bone marrow, gut, skin, liver, kidneys, brain and gonads.

We must always remember that our duty to patients is to help and not to harm them, and that a properly designed clinical experiment aims to do this and not simply to obtain information for its own sake.

Combination chemotherapy

It is theoretically possible that, by combining cytotoxic drugs, their anti-tumour effect will be additive or even synergistic while their side-effects are not. This can be achieved in part by choosing drugs all of which are known to be toxic to the tumour but which have different major side-effects. Vincristine, for example, may be profitably combined with cyclophosphamide; the major side-effect of vincristine is neurotoxicity while cyclophosphamide is mainly toxic to the bone marrow. An extension of this approach is that since different cytotoxic agents act at different sites in the cell, and at different parts of the cell cycle, their combination may in some way be synergistic and thus partly overcome problems of drug resistance.

In clinical practice this should result in higher remission rates and longer remission durations than can be achieved with single agents; and this has proved to be true, at least in some drug-sensitive malignancies such as Hodgkin's disease and acute leukaemia.

A criticism of combination chemotherapy is that one cannot be certain that a tumour is sensitive to all the drugs in the combination, so that at times the patient may incur a needless amount of toxicity. At present there is no satisfactory way of predicting the sensitivity of human tumours to any particular drug, and the choice of drugs for combination in the clinic has to be made on the basis of past experience. Some empirical rules have been proposed:

1. The treatment must be tolerable for the patient.
2. The drugs in a combination should be active against the tumour when used alone.
3. As far as possible, each drug should have a different major side-effect.
4. Attempts to exploit kinetic differences in the cell cycle between the tumour and the normal tissues should be made though these are not always successful.

Adjuvant chemotherapy

Adjuvant chemotherapy means the planned addition of chemotherapy to treatment with surgery, radiotherapy or both modes of treatment. There are two kinds of approach. The first is to use chemotherapy initially to facilitate some other kind of subsequent treatment. Examples are the use of nitrogen mustard for the rapid relief of spinal cord compression by a tumour. This can be followed by laminectomy and radiotherapy. Similarly, large tumours in the head and neck which are involving vital structures can be made transiently to shrink with chemotherapy after which radiotherapy or surgery may be easier.

The second and more important application of adjuvant chemotherapy is where it is used after surgery or radiotherapy to prevent the development of clinically detectable metastases and so to increase the disease-free life of the patient. The best examples of this form of treatment come from the management of children's tumours such as Ewing's tumour, Wilms' tumour and rhabdomyosarcoma. In all these cancers the major therapeutic problem is not local tumour control but the subsequent development of distant metastases which kill the patient.

The principles of the second type of adjuvant chemotherapy

remain the same, irrespective of the type of tumour. The treatment is given at a time when the patient is apparently free of tumour which has been removed surgically, irradiated or treated with a combination of the two sorts of therapy; and its aim is to eradicate microscopical metastases. It follows that before adjuvant chemotherapy is introduced into any treatment programme, two criteria must be satisfied. First the tumour must have been shown to be sensitive to a particular regime of chemotherapy in patients with measurable tumour. The second is that the group of patients with apparently localised disease must be significantly at risk for the development of clinically evident metastases if local treatment only is given.

As mentioned previously, these criteria are satisfied by some children's tumours. In Wilms' tumour, for example, a survival rate of 50 per cent has been reported for children with localised disease. Children who died did so mainly from lung metastases. This situation has been changed by the addition of chemotherapy so that the overall 10-year survival rate in Wilms' tumour may be as high as 80 per cent. In Ewing's tumour, only about 10 per cent of children treated locally are long-term survivors, but studies in which adjuvant chemotherapy has been used have demonstrated significantly increased survival.

Other tumours in which adjuvant chemotherapy is attracting attention are breast cancer, testicular teratoma, medulloblastoma, and ependymoma; it seems likely that, as better drug schedules are developed, this form of treatment will be increasingly applied.

From a kinetic point of view, adjuvant chemotherapy is particularly attractive since the chance of eradicating very small numbers of tumour cells is theoretically possible with the drugs already available; the chance of killing all the cells in a tumour which is clinically or radiologically obvious is far smaller. But what makes adjuvant chemotherapy somewhat unattractive is the need to overtreat some patients who will not develop metastases for the sake of those who will. At present there is no way of predicting which patients are definitely at risk for relapse after apparently curative local therapy, and it is here that the chemotherapist may hope that work on tumour index substances such as oncofetal antigens and hormones may provide the help that is needed.

In some circles it has become fashionable to suggest that adjuvant chemotherapy is going to be the means of controlling many common cancers such as those of the colon, rectum or lung. Such an approach is clearly naïve until better chemotherapy is developed, since no chemotherapy is yet available to which these tumours have consistently been shown to be sensitive. Furthermore to adopt such a view is to ignore the fact that failure to control tumours locally is still a significant part of the problem, that metastases are frequently not microscopic but may be very large and that secondary deposits, however small, may be chemoresistant or inaccessible to cytotoxic drugs. For many common tumours it is plain that we need better drugs and not simply better ways of using them.

SOME SELECTED EXAMPLES OF THE DRUG TREATMENT OF SPECIFIC TUMOURS

Three important questions concerning the chemosensitivity of tumours to drugs need to be considered. First, does the tumour consistently respond to chemotherapy? Second, does a response mean that life is prolonged? Third, does chemotherapy improve the quality of the patient's life? In some cases the answer is yes to all three questions. Hodgkin's disease provides a very good example. In other cases, although the tumour responds to chemotherapy by becoming smaller it is uncertain that life is prolonged by this. Neuroblastoma provides an example of this; there is no real evidence that children with widespread tumour live any longer as a result of drug treatment although there is little doubt that the quality of life is improved by treatment and this is important both for the child and his family. In the case of some tumours quality of life may be improved in the absence of any measurable evidence of tumour regression. An example is the relief of liver pain due to deposits of colonic tumours in patients treated with 5-fluorouracil.

Tables 1–5 summarise the current status of chemotherapy for a selection of tumours. It can be seen that there is no room for complacency since in general it is the rare tumours which are sensitive to drugs and the common ones which are not. The one major exception is breast cancer but even here many responses last less than a year, and there is as yet no evidence that anyone is cured by chemotherapy even when it is used as an adjuvant following surgery.

Table 1

Tumours in which chemotherapy may be curative or contribute to cure when used with other sorts of treatment

- Choriocarcinoma (in women)
- Burkitt's lymphoma
- Acute lymphoblastic leukaemia in children
- Hodgkin's disease
- Wilms' tumour
- Embryonal rhabdomyosarcoma

Table 2

Tumours which are frequently sensitive to cytotoxic drugs and where remissions are often obtained and life is prolonged

- Non-Hodgkin's lymphomas
- Breast carcinoma
- Testicular tumours
- Acute lymphoblastic leukaemia

Table 3

Tumours which are sometimes sensitive to cytotoxic drugs, where remissions occur and life is sometimes prolonged

- Ovarian carcinoma
- Myeloma
- Osteogenic sarcoma
- Soft tissue sarcomas
- Oat cell carcinoma of the bronchus

Table 4

Tumours where, although response to chemotherapy occurs, it is uncertain whether life is prolonged

- Colorectal carcinoma
- Melanoma
- Bladder carcinoma
- Chronic myeloid leukaemia
- Squamous cell carcinoma of the skin
- Neuroblastoma
- Carcinoma of the cervix
- Carcinoma of the larynx

TABLE 5

Tumours in which a response to
chemotherapy is seldom seen
and life is not prolonged

> Carcinoma of the stomach
> Carcinoma of the pancreas
> Chondrosarcoma
> Mesothelioma

THE USE OF CHEMOTHERAPY FOR SELECTED TUMOURS

Leukaemia

The major advances have been made in acute lymphoblastic leukaemia (ALL) of childhood; first single agents and then combination chemotherapy of increasing complexity has steadily improved remission rates and length of survival.

Success has not only been due to chemotherapy but also to the parallel development of better supportive treatment with whole blood platelet and granulocytic transfusions, broad spectrum antibiotics and possible protective isolation facilities. The major non-haematological complication of ALL – leukaemia meningopathy – has been greatly reduced by the introduction of planned early radiotherapy to the central nervous system; finally, leukaemia centres staffed by workers with a special interest in the disease have collected patients together, so increasing the rate at which problems can be identified and tackled, and information disseminated. The development of multicentre co-operative clinical groups has raised the overall standard of leukaemia treatment in the community so that the child with ALL should now have a 50 per cent chance of surviving disease-free for five years. Adults and children over the age of 12 with ALL fare less well and tend to relapse within one to two years of starting treatment. It is here that further effort directed at a better understanding of the biology of the disease and designing more eradicative chemotherapy needs to be directed.

Acute myeloblastic leukaemia (AML), on the other hand, still presents an immense challenge. Only about 60 per cent of patients treated with a variety of drug combinations achieve remission, and few of those individuals survive for longer than one year. To be effective, drug treatment often needs to be pushed to the limits of toxicity. The crux of the problem is the very small degree of tumour cell selectivity shown by the drugs most active against AML. What is needed here is drugs that are less toxic to the patient and more active against the tumour; but until these are available clinical studies continue with the available agents in which the emphasis is on devising combinations and sequences of drugs that exploit such differences as exist between the proliferation kinetics of the tumour and the normal host tissues.

Lymphomas

In Hodgkin's disease the role of chemotherapy is fairly well defined. It is used in three main situations; as an adjuvant before radiotherapy when very large masses of tumour require shrinkage; in newly diagnosed patients with widely disseminated disease and as an adjuvant following radiotherapy in high-risk patients. Combination chemotherapy has made an enormous difference here. Complete remission rates of over 70 per cent can be achieved with combinations compared with rates of about 20 per cent when the drugs are used singly. The majority of patients now live more than five years from the start of chemotherapy and it is probable that some are cured. Those who relapse can be retreated, since the tumour is sensitive to many cytotoxic drugs.

In the non-Hodgkin's lymphomas response to chemotherapy is variable and largely depends upon the type of tumour. The relatively 'benign' follicular lymphomas respond well to chemotherapy whereas the most aggressive diffuse poorly differentiated tumours are less chemo-responsive. There is no doubt, however, that chemotherapy is often effective in this group of tumours and patients whose tumours respond live longer.

Breast cancer

Responses to combination chemotherapy in breast cancer are frequent and sometimes complete. Many drugs can be used and no particular combination can be regarded as a 'best buy'. An average response rate for most combinations would be about 60 per cent. Metastatic disease in some sites responds more favourably than in others. Thus, responses in soft tissue are common whereas bone metastases respond poorly and are better treated by endocrine therapy. It is important to stress that chemotherapy and endocrine therapy should not be regarded as competing treatments but rather as complementary to one another; the best treatment for an individual patient depending upon her age, her menstrual status, the time interval between primary treatment and relapse, and the site of relapse.

Recently many studies of adjuvant chemotherapy have been launched in patients whose disease remains localised at presentation and is apparently completely removed by surgery. Preliminary results suggest that chemotherapy prolongs the duration of first remission in pre-menopausal women, but does not do so significantly in post-menopausal patients. It is too early to say whether any patient has been cured by adjuvant chemotherapy and much time will need to pass before we know the answer to this question. Until then the use of adjuvant chemotherapy must be regarded as experimental and oncologists need to resist pressures, both professional and public, to regard it as an established method of treatment of breast cancer.

Cancer in childhood

Cancer ranks second only to accidents as a cause of death in British children. The crux of the problem is that local treatment with surgery and radiotherapy seldom leads to cure since most children's tumours have spread beyond the primary site when the patient is first seen. Fortunately, many of these tumours are chemo-sensitive and the use of adjuvant chemotherapy has greatly improved survival and has definitely contributed to cure in some patients.

Early success with adjuvant chemotherapy was achieved in

Wilms' tumour, a highly malignant growth in the kidney of children. Here the cure rate has been increased from about 30 per cent to 80 per cent by the use of chemotherapy. Similar encouraging results are now being seen with rhabdomyosarcoma, a tumour of muscle, and in some tumours of bone. There is one childhood tumour where chemotherapy has made little, if any, impact, on survival and this is neuroblastoma which accounts for about nine per cent of childhood cancer. At present attempts are being made to combine chemotherapy and radiotherapy in high doses, but it is too early to say whether these approaches will improve matters.

Lung cancer

Less than 10 per cent of all patients with lung cancer are cured by surgery or radiotherapy, and the majority of affected individuals die of metastases. Oat cell carcinomas are particularly malignant and most patients have clinically obvious metastases at or within a few months of presentation. There is about a 45 per cent incidence of bone marrow metastases detectable at presentation which almost certainly means that their true incidence is higher. For these reasons it is clear that lung cancer (and oat cell carcinoma in particular) is usually a generalised disease at presentation so that efforts directed at achieving better control of the primary tumour are unlikely greatly to improve prognosis.

Several drugs are known to produce regressions in lung cancer and their use in combination is now being examined in conjunction with surgery and radiotherapy. Earlier experience with single agents failed to show any benefit when cyclophosphamide or nitrogen mustard were combined with surgery; recently the use of combination chemotherapy has produced responses in patients with oat cell carcinoma and there is evidence that patients in whom response occurs, live longer than those whose tumours do not respond. Very few meaningful responses have been seen in patients with adenocarcinoma or squamous cell carcinoma, and it is still questionable whether many patients with these tumours should receive chemotherapy at all. The fact remains that the judicious use of chemotherapy in selected patients with lung cancer is now proving beneficial.

Other tumours

Many other tumours will respond to chemotherapy. For example there is now good evidence that the rare testicular teratomas frequently respond to combinations of drugs and that these, when properly combined with surgery and radiotherapy, contribute to the cure of patients. Malignant melanoma responds to several drugs, but prolongation of life is not common, although there may be improvement of quality of life. A similar pattern is seen with other tumours such as those of the cervix, bladder, stomach and colon where the best that we can expect is short-term palliation.

These gloomy results spotlight the need for new and better drugs as well as the need for a deeper understanding of the biology of malignant and normal tissue. At present clinical cancer chemotherapy is frequently ineffective and often unpleasant for the patient; although gains in the understanding of the biology of tumours and normal tissues have contributed to the development of safer and more effective treatment, much of what is done in the clinic is empirically based on past clinical experience and is likely to remain so for a long time. Furthermore, no amount of scientific expertise will make up for a sympathetic and understanding approach to the patient, or the ability to explain his disease and its treatment to him.

2. Care of Patients receiving Anti-tumour Drugs

by ELSPETH WARK SRN, FETC

Anti-tumour drug therapy is a continuously expanding field of cancer treatment. This form of treatment is no longer used only as a measure to palliate patients with extensive disease, but is used with surgery and radiotherapy as part of curative treatment in primary disease. Knowledge of the biological and psychological effects of cancer chemotherapy on the patient is essential.

Patients will react to their disease and treatment as they individually inter-react in society. The position in the community that each patient identifies as theirs depends on their sex, age, social background, education and job specification. This concept will inevitably be under stress when malignant disease is suspected. The diagnosis of cancer carries the threat of shortened life and its connotations to a young adult starting his first job, the mother with young children, the middle-aged father with a mortgage or the elderly grandmother will require assessment on an individual basis. The needs of these patients, whether physical or emotional, are difficult to separate and the care and support the nurse can give must involve the whole family unit. Recognition of the behavioural responses to anxiety and stress will enhance the development of an understanding, trusting relationship between the patient and nurse. Encouraging the patient to put into words his feelings about having cancer and being sick, and his immediate concerns regarding treatment as well as his worries about the future, reduce anxiety and tension for both the patient and the nurse. The assessment of the social and physical status of the patient needs to be undertaken before the prescribed treatment is commenced. Any nursing problems can be ascertained and acted upon immediately thus assuring some release of the anxiety and fear in the patient.

Close liaison between physicians and nurses responsible for

CARE FOLLOWING ANTI-TUMOUR DRUGS

patients receiving anti-tumour drugs is of prime importance. The major biochemical, haematological and radiological changes which may occur with these treatments need to be communicated to the nurses concerned so that they may observe and report if the slightest symptom or sign of change is noted. Such changes in the patient's condition may require modification of the treatment protocol and the nursing objectives. This exchange of information will ensure the best possible care for the patient as well as contributing to the physician's evaluation of the drugs' effects. Prior knowledge of the aims of the treatment protocol which should include the rationale for the use of the particular drugs, the dose and route of administration, the known or expected side-effects, the specimens required and procedures planned, will alleviate the anxiety of the nurse dealing with the unknown; it will also allow the nurse to convey confidence and competence to the patient when giving care.

Prior to the commencement of treatment, a variety of investigations are carried out in order to evaluate the current physiological state of the patient and the extent of the disease. The pace of these investigations is often rapid and exhausting to the patient who becomes physically and emotionally tired. The patient may require repeated explanation of these examinations and procedures; he will want to know what is to happen and also how he may feel at the completion of the procedure. By carefully planning her care, the nurse can ensure that the investigations are organised promptly and efficiently, and thus reduce to a minimum worry and discomfort for the patient.

INVESTIGATIONS

1. Measurement of height and weight: most drug doses are calculated on the body surface area using a nomogram or on each kilogram of body weight.
2. Full blood count: haemoglobin, white cell count with differentials and platelets are the most important, although blood chemistry will also be assessed.
3. Kidney function test: there are a great variety of these

investigations, the most common being a 24-hour urine collection for creatinine clearance or blood plasma levels following administration of EDTA (ethylene diamine tetra-acetic acid) using a chromium^{51} marker.
4. Liver function test: these are usually serum alkaline phosphatase, glutamic pyruvic transaminase (GPT) and, if necessary, serum bilirubin.
5. Bone marrow biopsy: this is performed if the peripheral blood count is abnormal or if the natural history of the particular malignant disease may involve the bone marrow at some stage.

The following examinations may be carried out to detect the extent of the disease and be used for an objective assessment of the effect of treatment on the malignant tumour.

1. X-rays and tomograms of various sites
2. Skeletal survey
3. Bone, liver, spleen and brain scan
4. Lymphogram and intravenous pyelogram
5. Ultrasound of specified sites
6. Electrocardiogram: this is carried out when anti-tumour drugs known to affect the heart are to be used.

TECHNIQUES OF ADMINISTRATION

The anti-tumour drugs now in use can be administered in a variety of ways: intravenously, orally, intramuscularly, intra-arterially, subcutaneously, and intrathecally. Many drugs are packaged to be given in a specific way and it is necessary for the nurse to check the literature accompanying the drugs to ascertain the correct route of administration.

There are different methods of administering anti-tumour drugs in the treatment of malignant disease and their effects on normal and malignant tissues are also different. They are:

(a) *Low dose continuous therapy using one drug*: this method leads to high toxic effects on the body and rapid development of tumour resistance to the drug. It is seldom used at the present time.

(b) *Low dose combination therapy over an extended period*: this technique produces accumulating toxic effects especially on the bone marrow. Tumour resistance to these drugs is slower to develop.

(c) *High dose intermittent therapy with one drug*: this method produces few toxic effects, but resistance of the tumour to the drug develops quickly.

(d) *High dose intermittent combination therapy*: this technique produces fewer side-effects and resistance of the tumour to the drugs is very slow to develop. The drugs are given over a short period of time and the bone marrow is allowed to recover before the next treatment is given. This is the most common method used at the present time.

(e) *Arterial infusion*: the artery which supplies the area of the tumour is cannulated and the drug infused over a period of time. The drug reaches the tumour in high concentrations but then enters the general circulation, producing systemic toxicity.

(f) *Regional perfusion*: perfusion requires temporary isolation of the part from the circulatory system and the part isolated is then maintained by a pump and oxygenator. Only the extremities can be perfused adequately and this method is seldom in use today.

(g) *Combined with radiotherapy and surgery*: anti-tumour drug therapy is now being given before or after surgery and/or radiotherapy as part of continuous treatment. Although radiotherapy and cancer chemotherapy do not have the same action on the cells, they do have similar side-effects and are not commonly used together at the same time.

Although the drugs will have been prescribed by the medical staff, their administration is increasingly becoming the responsibility of the trained nurse. A knowledge of the drugs, their mode of action and expected drug effect, both toxic and therapeutic, is of paramount importance. Because of the interaction of drugs and their stability in solution it is important that information regarding the storage, diluents, available strengths and any other relevant information necessary to ensure the correct and most effective administration of the drug be available to the nurse.

Close attention must be paid to intravenous infusions. The rate of infusion must be carefully monitored and the use of a self-regulating infusion pump will ensure accuracy. In patients whose pulmonary or cardiac function is impaired, too rapid an infusion can result in pulmonary oedema. In patients whose intake is poor, too slow an infusion can result in poor kidney function or dehydration. Coupled with this is the need to administer the drug in the prescribed time to be of the most effective therapeutic effect.

Since the nurse spends more time with the patient than other members of the health care team, she has a better opportunity to know the patient and be familiar with his physical and emotional condition on a daily basis. The nurse may be the first to recognise even the most subtle signs of either drug toxicity or therapeutic effect by her own observation or by the patient being able to talk more easily to her than to the physician. Many patients receiving anti-tumour drug therapy may feel well and being mobile on the ward appear to require little nursing care. Their appearance and activity can be deceptive and careful attention must be given to them. When the nursing care plan is being formulated, the nurse's knowledge of the toxic effects of the drugs need to be incorporated into it so that complications which may ensue can be distinguished from those that may arise from the disease process. The toxicity of anti-tumour drug treatment will mainly affect those areas of the body where normal cell activity is high and the nurse's observation of these systems may ensure early recognition and prompt action to minimise the effects.

THE BONE MARROW

Bone marrow depression which will cause anaemia, thrombocytopenia and leucopenia, is probably the most severe toxic manifestation of anti-tumour drugs. Nearly all the drugs in common use will affect the bone marrow in varying degrees.

Leucopenia

A low white cell count will inevitably increase the risk of infection, but it may manifest itself in an atypical manner. The patient's skin will need examination for open or reddened areas that could be potential sites for infection. His mouth and throat should also be inspected daily with a torch for signs of local infection. The temperature is taken at least four hourly or more frequently if the patient becomes lethargic, appears flushed or feels warm to the touch. The temperature can rise rapidly from 37°C to 40°C in a few hours. If the nurse is alert to the danger of local infection, septicaemia may be avoided by immediate and effective antibiotic therapy. The nurse has a responsibility to ensure that the leucopenic patient is nursed away from possible sources of infection and occasionally it may be necessary to place the patient in a pathogen-reduced environment such as a 'life-island' or special isolation unit.

Thrombocytopenia

A low platelet count increases the danger of bleeding. The initial sites of bleeding may be from the gums, nasal passages, the urinary or gastro-intestinal tracts. The appearance of petechiae on areas of the body unexplained by trauma are critical signs. The nurse should routinely check these areas for initial signs of bleeding including the testing of urine and faeces. The patient needs to be aware of the importance of immediately reporting any bleeding from his nose or gums. The nurse can recommend the use of a soft toothbrush and encourage male patients to use an electric razor for shaving. Intramuscular injections should also be avoided when the platelet count is low. If the platelet count falls to a critical level and warning signs of bleeding occur, a platelet transfusion or fresh blood transfusion will be given.

Anaemia

Due to the longevity of red cells, the symptoms of anaemia are slower to develop than those of leucopenia and thrombocytopenia. The resultant lethargy, fatigue and dyspnoea may require a blood transfusion.

GASTRO-INTESTINAL TRACT

Mouth

Before anti-tumour drug therapy is commenced, the nurse should examine the patient's mouth for any inflammation, infection and observe the general state of oral hygiene. Dentures should be checked for fit and if there are problems, the patient should be seen by the dentist before therapy is commenced. The nurse must emphasise the importance of good oral hygiene and teach the patient proper care of his mouth in order to reduce possible reactions. Some anti-tumour drugs have a toxic effect which leads to mouth ulceration. One of the earliest signs of possible ulceration is that the patient may comment on an increased sensitivity to hot and cold food and a painful or burning sensation from citric or spicy foods. Symptoms usually start with dryness of the mouth, a burning sensation of the lips or a line of erythema and oedema along the muco-cutaneous junction of the lip with shallow ulcers appearing. If this stomatitis is recognised early, extensive ulceration, severe dysphagia and secondary infection may be avoided by prompt action in reporting them to the medical team. Some discomfort may be inevitable, but frequent mouthwashes using glycothymoline, soda bicarbonate and half-strength hydrogen peroxide, although unpalatable, will keep the mouth clean. Gentian violet is excellent when painted on ulceration and also aids in the prevention of fungal infections. The patient's diet will need careful planning to avoid highly seasoned or acid foods and to encourage high protein intake to aid in the recovery of normal cells.

Stomach

Anorexia, nausea and vomiting, which are associated with most anti-tumour drugs, may be caused by numerous physiological changes, such as irritability and increased tension on the walls of the stomach and duodenum or irritation of the mucosa which stimulates the vomiting centre in the medulla with subsequent anorexia. Anorexia and nausea can often be tolerated by the

CARE FOLLOWING ANTI-TUMOUR DRUGS

patient due to the short period it is experienced. Vomiting, on the other hand, can lead to serious fluid and electrolyte imbalance. The nurse caring for patients who are nauseated and vomiting can help reduce these effects by using well-tried methods and her ingenuity. The patient should be sat up in a comfortable position, given mouth care before and after meals and the bed placed in good ventilation away from sights, sounds and smells which may exacerbate the condition. Meals need to be small, attractively served to tempt the appetite and given with greater frequency. Waves of nausea may be lessened by deep breathing and sipping effervescent fluids or sucking ice. The usual methods taken for any patient who is vomiting are proper positioning to prevent inhalation of vomit, noting the time of onset in relation to the intake of food or administration of the drugs, and the frequency of the episodes. Anti-emetics are usually prescribed and given prophylactically before and after administration of anti-tumour drugs which are known to cause vomiting. The nurse needs to maintain an accurate fluid balance chart and to be prompt in reporting signs of electrolyte imbalance and dehydration.

Bowel

Diarrhoea, like vomiting, may lead to dehydration and electrolyte imbalance since large amounts of water are lost. It is essential that basic nursing duties such as emptying bedpans are carried out by experienced nurses who can assess the colour and consistency and recognise the early signs of toxicity and dehydration. As the normal bowel pattern of the patient is known by the nurse who assessed the patient on admission, early bowel changes will be noted and treatment with anti-diarrhoeal drugs initiated early. Some control may also be effected by a low residue and bland diet.

SKIN AND HAIR

Alopecia can occur with some of the anti-tumour drugs in use and the patient should be aware of this before treatment commences. The psychological distress that female and male patients experience can often be severe and must never be underestimated. To aid them in coming to terms with this effect, a properly fitted wig should be ordered before treatment commences. Once this has been done, the patient will feel that those who are caring for him have acknowledged the problem and taken practical steps to alleviate it. Patients can be truthfully reassured that their hair will grow again at the end of treatment or in some cases, even before the end of treatment. Head tourniquets, used originally in the hope of preventing hair loss, have now been shown to have no real value. Epilation of body hair will also occur in varying degrees.

Special attention should be paid to the pressure areas of patients confined to bed. Frequent and effective skin care must be given to prevent breakdown. Positioning, turning and assisting the patient in and out of bed to avoid trauma is important and the use of sheepskins, foam pads and ripple mattresses may be helpful.

Nail growth is retarded and with some anti-tumour drugs there may be pigmentation. Exfoliative dermatitis, erythema especially in areas of previous radiotherapy, and pigmentation of the skin are rare but reported side-effects of some drugs. The nurse should, however, be aware of the possibility of these occurrences to ease the patient's mind by distinguishing these symptoms from those of the disease process.

URINARY SYSTEM

Kidney

Nephrotoxicity may result from the use of some anti-tumour drugs. It can also result from the poor excretion of uric acid, a by-product of large cell death due to the anti-tumour drug activity. Maintaining careful intake and output records and observing the frequency and colour of urine are all important nursing duties. Because the drugs are primarily excreted through the kidney, accurate records must be kept as poor kidney function may cause increased absorption of the drug into the blood, thereby increasing the toxic effects on the other systems of the body.

Bladder

A very painful chemical cystitis may develop due to close proximity of the drugs to the bladder mucosa. This effect can be prevented by encouraging a high fluid intake aiding a high fluid output. If cystitis occurs, treatment can consist of antibiotics, antispasmodics, intravenous fluids and diuretics.

GONADS

Many anti-tumour drugs have been reported to induce amenorrhoea and temporary sterility in men and women. Their mutagenic properties, if any, are not known, although spontaneous abortions and abnormal fetuses have occurred. Patients of childbearing age should be informed of these unknown effects and advice given about forms of contraception, which should be continued for the duration of treatment and for at least 12 months following, to allow time for gonad recovery.

NERVOUS SYSTEM

Most anti-tumour drugs do not cross the blood/brain barrier in therapeutically effective doses, but small amounts are sufficient to produce toxic effects on the central nervous system. The symptoms may be nausea and vomiting, general depression, lack of concentration, interference with the autonomic nervous system and peripheral neuritis.

Nausea and vomiting can be dealt with as described earlier. General depression is usually treated with anti-depressant drugs, tranquillisers and supportive emotional care. The vinca alkaloids may cause interference with the function of the autonomic nervous system which can lead to severe constipation. To prevent impaction of faeces due to an atonic large bowel, daily checking of bowel function and prophylactic treatment with a wetting agent and a mild aperient should be commenced with treatment. Decreased or non-functioning of the large bowel, if not reported by the patient or noticed by the nurse, can result in serious impaction, obstruction and even perforation of the colon due to the already affected mucosa by other anti-tumour drugs. It should be noted that constipation and impaction appears in the upper colon and not in the rectum so digital inspection may not reveal the early signs of the problem. The vinca alkaloids may also cause peripheral neuritis, usually noted initially as tingling in the extremities and on occasion in the parotid glands. Other signs may be lack of co-ordination, loss of balance or changes in gait. These changes may be so subtle that only the nurse noting the activity level of the patient on a daily basis would recognise the change. These changes must be reported immediately as this condition is progressive and will lead to permanent muscle damage if treatment is not interrupted.

CARDIAC AND PULMONARY SYSTEMS

Cardio-toxicity is a side-effect of a small number of anti-tumour drugs in current use. Before the commencement of treatment, an electrocardiogram should be carried out to act as a baseline when further checks are undertaken; the nurse can monitor the pulse for irregularities in the rate and volume. Effects on the lungs can lead to pulmonary fibrosis, and the nurse may detect early signs by observing dyspnoea and dry unproductive coughing. Treatment is the administration of steroids and antibiotics if superimposed infection occurs.

Caring for patients receiving anti-tumour drugs requires full use of the knowledge, judgement, skills and understanding of the trained nurse. It is important, that basic nursing procedures and observations be undertaken by experienced nurses allocated to the patient so that the nurse is then able to interpret any relevant changes in the patient's condition. As well as being a constant and thorough observer for the effects of drugs, the nurse must give physical and emotional support to the patient. Nursing the cancer patient receiving anti-tumour drugs is not easy: it is exacting, physically tiring, at times discouraging, but always calling upon all the nurse's resources. It is challenging, intriguing and rewarding for the informed nurse who, as part of the caring team, is able to meet the complex needs of the patient.

CLASSIFICATION AND USES OF ANTI-TUMOUR AGENTS

	Specific Information	Side-effects	Nursing Implication
1. ANTI METABOLITES			
cytosine arabinoside (Ara-C)	1 Metabolised by liver Hepatotoxicity 2 Excreted by kidneys 3 Crosses blood/brain barrier	1 Bone marrow depression 2 Stomatitis 3 Nausea and vomiting at high doses 4 Hyperuricaemia	—potential infection, bleeding —oral hygiene, bland diet —dietary control, encourage fluids —observe urinary output
5-fluorouracil (5FU)	1 Darkening of veins with prolonged use especially of dark-skinned patients	1 Bone marrow depression 2 Stomatitis 3 Nausea and vomiting 4 Diarrhoea 5 Some alopecia	—potential infection, bleeding —oral hygiene, bland diet —dietary control encourage fluids —diet, kaolin compounds —arrange for wig Protect from light Avoid extravasation

	Specific Information	Side-effects	Nursing Implication
1. ANTI METABOLITES			
6-mercaptopurine (6MP)	1 Increased potency when used with allopurinol (due to delay in its metabolism)	1 Bone marrow depression 2 Stomatitis 3 Nausea and vomiting 4 Diarrhoea 5 Liver dysfunction	—potential infection, bleeding —oral hygiene, bland diet —dietary control, encourage fluids —diet, kaolin compounds —observe for jaundice bilirubin in urine
methotrexate (MTX)	1 Folic acid antagonist: Leucovorin rescue at 24 hours after drug dose if: a. MTX infused b. given IM c. impaired renal function 2 Incompatible with sulphonamides 3 Nephro and hepatotoxic at high doses 4 Avoid use with salicylates	1 Bone marrow depression 2 Stomatitis 3 Nausea and vomiting 4 Diarrhoea 5 Skin rash 6 Photosensitivity 7 Cystitis	—potential infection, bleeding —oral hygiene, bland diet —dietary control, encourage fluids —diet, kaolin compounds —calamine lotion or steroid cream —keep IV away from sunlight —encourage fluids, observe urinary output

2. ALKYLATING AGENTS	Specific Information	Side-effects	Nursing Implication
cyclophosphamide (Endoxana)	1 Excreted via kidneys 2 Immunosuppressant 3 Body 'flushes' at time of injection	1 Bone marrow depression 2 Stomatitis 3 Nausea and vomiting 4 Alopecia 5 Chemical cystitis 6 Alteration in taste	—potential infection, bleeding —oral hygiene, bland diet —dietary control, encourage fluids —arrange for wig —high fluid intake and adequate output essential, forced diuresis above 3.5g doses —use of flavourisers
busulphan (Myleran)	1 Has cumulative effect at about 300mg WBC may fall and not recover 2 Excreted by kidneys	1 Bone marrow depression 2 Gynaecomastia, amenorrhoea 3 Skin pigmentation 4 Irreversible pulmonary fibrosis	—potential infection, bleeding —inform patient —inform patient —steroids usually given
chlorambucil (Leukeran)	Slow onset	1 Bone marrow depression 2 Nausea and vomiting } at high doses. 3 Dermatitis	—potential infection, bleeding —encourage fluids, dietary control —calamine lotion or steroid cream

2. ALKYLATING AGENTS	Specific Information	Side-effects	Nursing Implication
L-Phenylalanine Mustard (melphalan)	1 No acute toxicity 2 Slow metabolism	1 Bone marrow depression 2 Nausea 3 Alopecia	—potential infection, bleeding —dietary control, encourage fluids —arrange for wig
mustine (Nitrogen Mustard)	1 Rapid acting 2 Darkening of veins with prolonged use	1 Bone marrow depression 2 Severe nausea and vomiting	—potential infection, bleeding —dietary control, encourage fluids Beware of skin and eye contamination Avoid extravasation
Triethylene Triphosphoramide (thiotepa)	1 Slow cumulative response 2 Excreted by kidneys	1 Bone marrow depression 2 Some nausea and vomiting 3 Allergic reaction, headache, fever 4 G.I. perforation 5 Mild anaemia	—potential infection, bleeding —dietary control, encourage fluids —regular nursing observations —watch for abdominal pain —adequate rest

	Specific Information	Side-effects	Nursing Implication
3. NATURAL PRODUCTS			
Adriamycin (doxyrubicin)	1 Antibiotic derivative 2 Metabolised by liver	1 Bone marrow depression 2 Stomatitis 3 Nausea, vomiting 4 Diarrhoea 5 Alopecia 6 Fever 7 Red urine up to 12 days 8 Cardiotoxocity 9 Thrombophlebitis	—potential infection, bleeding —oral hygiene, bland diet —dietary control, encourage fluids —diet, kaolin compounds —arrange for wig —inform patient —ECG essential pre-dose, observation of pulse —encourage mobility Avoid extravasation
actinomycin D (Cosmegen)	1 Antibiotic derivative 2 **If previous recent radiation, drug may reactivate site of radiation** 3 Nephrotoxic and hepatotoxic	1 Bone marrow depression 2 Stomatitis 3 Nausea, vomiting 4 Diarrhoea 5 Alopecia 6 Skin pigmentation 7 Anorexia 8 Mental depression 9 Anaphylaxis – rare	—potential infection, bleeding —oral hygiene, bland diet —dietary control, encourage fluids —diet, kaolin compounds —arrange for wig —inform patient —appetising food —psychological support Avoid extravasation

3. NATURAL PRODUCTS	Specific Information	Side-effects	Nursing Implication
L-asparaginase	1 Enzyme which binds asparagine 2 Do *not* shake vial use clear solution only Bayer makes Porton 3 Reversible encephalopathy Reversible hepatotoxicity	1 Nausea, vomiting 50% 2 Malaise 3 Anaphylaxis 4 Hypoglycaemia 5 Hypoalbuminaemia	—dietary control, encourage fluids —psychological support —emergency equipment ready hydrocortisone and Piriton ready —collection of specimens —collection of specimens
platinum	Colloid of platinum	1 Bone marrow depression 2 Severe nausea, vomiting 3 Diarrhoea 4 Renal failure	—potential infection, bleeding —dietary control, encourage fluids —diet, kaolin compounds —forced diuresis for high doses, observe urea and creatinine

Drug	Notes	Side effects	Nursing care
daunorubicin (Rubidomycin)	1 Antibiotic derivative 2 Contra-indicated where infection present	1 Bone marrow depression 2 Stomatitis 3 Nausea, vomiting, fever 4 Alopecia 5 Red urine 6 Abdominal pain, phlebitis 7 Congestive cardiac failure	—potential infection, bleeding —oral hygiene, bland diet —dietary control, encourage fluids —arrange for wig —inform patient —ECG essential pre-dose, observation and reporting of symptoms Avoid extravasation Protect from light
bleomycin	1 Antibiotic derivative 2 Has very little effect on bone marrow 3 Contra-indicated if pulmonary abnormalities	1 Stomatitis 2 Nausea and vomiting 3 Alopecia 4 Tumour pain 5 Macular pain 6 Anaphylaxis 3–5 hrs after high doses 7 Pulmonary fibrosis	—oral hygiene, bland diet —dietary control, encourage fluids —arrange for wig —administration of analgesia —observe patient, emergency equipment to hand —weekly chest X-ray If IM, lignocaine 1% plain added to relieve pain Avoid skin contamination

	Specific Information	Side-effects	Nursing Implication
3. NATURAL PRODUCTS			
mithramycin	1 Antibiotic derivative 2 Used for hypercalcaemia 3 Hepatic and nephrotoxic	1 Stomatitis 2 Nausea, vomiting, fever 3 Diarrhoea 4 Haemorrhagic-epistaxis 5 Hypocalcaemia (rare) 6 Headache, depression, drowsiness	—oral hygiene, bland diet —dietary control, encourage fluids —diet, kaolin compounds —stop bleeding, ice pack etc. —observe for increased neural and muscular excitability —inform patient and observe Avoid extravasation
Mitomycin-C	1 Antibiotic derivative 2 Nephrotoxic (rare)	1 Bone marrow depression 2 Stomatitis 3 Nausea, vomiting, fever 4 Alopecia 5 Paraesthesia 6 Pruritis	—potential infection, bleeding —oral hygiene, bland diet —dietary control, encourage fluids —arrange for wig —observe —anti-pruritic cream Avoid extravasation

vinblastine	1 Extracted from periwinkle rosea
	2 Profound leukopenia if cachexia or ulcerated areas of skin present
	3 Contra indicated where:
	  a. bacterial infection
	  b. leukopenia
	  c. impaired circulatory function in limbs
	4 Neurotoxic (rare)
		1 Bone marrow depression
		2 Nausea and vomiting
		3 Epilation
		4 Peripheral neuritis
		5 Headache, dizziness
		6 Constipation
			—potential infection, bleeding
			—dietary control, encourage fluids
			—arrange for wig
			—report symptoms, observe for numbness, ataxia
			—observe, give analgesics
			—mild aperient and wetting agent
			
			Avoid extravasation

vincristine (Oncovin)	1 Extracted from periwinkle rosea 2 Metabolised by liver 3 Neurotoxic	1 Stomatitis 2 Nausea and vomiting 3 Alopecia 4 Abdominal colic, constipation – upper colon impaction 5 Peripheral neuritis, tingling, ataxia, neuritic pain, paraesthesia 6 Dysuria, polyuria	—oral hygiene, bland diet —dietary control, encourage fluids —arrange for wig —mild aperient and wetting agent, prophylactically —warn patient and report symptoms immediately —observe urinary output Avoid extravasation or contamination of eye

4. OTHER AGENTS	Specific Information	Side-effects	Nursing Implication
hydroxyurea	1 Crosses blood/brain barrier	1 Bone marrow depression 2 Stomatitis 3 Nausea and vomiting 4 Diarrhoea 5 Anorexia 6 Alopecia (mild) 7 Erythema, rash, pruritus	—potential infection, bleeding —oral hygiene, bland diet —dietary control, encourage fluids —diet, kaolin compounds —arrange for wig —non-perfumed soaps, skin cleanliness If given as 24 hr infusion, ½ hourly observation owing to possibility of anaphylaxis.
procarbazine (Natulan)	1 Metabolised by liver 2 Excreted by kidneys 3 Crosses blood/brain barrier	1 Bone marrow depression 2 Nausea and vomiting 3 Alopecia 4 Mild CNS toxicity 5 MAO inhibitor	—potential infection, bleeding —dietary control, encourage fluids —arrange for wig —observe and report —no alcohol, cheese, Marmite, yoghurt, no sedatives, narcotics, tricyclic antidepressants, antihistamines

BIBLIOGRAPHY

Bouchard, R. and Owens, N. (1972). *Nursing Care of the Cancer Patient*. Mosby, St Louis, Ill.

Duncan Behnke, Helen (Ed.) (1973). *Guidelines for Comprehensive Nursing Care in Cancer*. Springer, New York.

Holz Peterson, Barbara and Kellog, Carolyn Jo (1976). *Current Practice in Oncological Nursing*. Vol. I. Mosby, St Louis, Ill.

Tiffany, Robert (1976). Nursing Care in Anti-tumour Drug Therapy. *Nursing Mirror 1 April*.

ACKNOWLEDGEMENT

This chapter is based on the article Nursing Care in Anti-tumour Drug Therapy by Robert Tiffany, and which appeared in the *Nursing Mirror*. The author is grateful to the Editor of *Nursing Mirror* for permission to adapt it.

3. Care of Patients receiving Hormonal Therapy

by GILLIAN DIGGORY SRN, RCNT

In reviewing the place of endocrine therapy in the management of malignant disease, this chapter will cover the types of tumour most commonly treated by hormones and steroids, the unwanted side-effects of treatment and the nurse's role in mitigating such side-effects. Physiological detail of endocrine secretion has been omitted, as it is adequately described in standard anatomy and physiology text books. Hormonal compounds can be used in the management of malignant disease because of their direct effect on tumour growth or as an adjuvant to other forms of therapy to enhance their effect. They may also be used indirectly to reduce the side-effects of other forms of therapy, e.g. the use of steroids to lessen cerebral oedema during cranial irradiation.

CANCER OF THE BREAST

One of the most common hormonal dependent tumours is cancer of the female breast. It is the target organ for a number of different hormones and in order to be able to comprehend the rationale for endocrine therapy it is important to understand where these hormones arise and their effect.

During each menstrual cycle there is a proliferation of the duct system and the stroma of fibrous and adipose tissue. This is followed by a partial regression of influencing hormones. During the first half of pregnancy the stroma and the duct system undergo a more extensive proliferation and yet another when lactation occurs. The hormones responsible for these changes are oestrogen, progesterone, prolactin, growth hormone and cortisone. Oestrogen will effect a change by the proliferation of the duct system and cause the nipple to thicken. Progesterone has no effect on its own, but in conjunction with oestrogen will cause glandular development in the alveoli. Prolactin is thought to stimulate lactation but this has not been firmly established, and it is thought that growth hormone, cortisone, and to some extent thyroxin, might also have an effect on breast tissue (see Fig. 3/1).

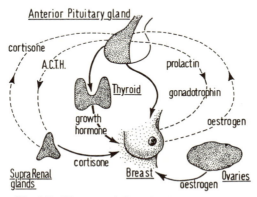

Fig. 3/1   Hormones influencing breast tumours
————— Direct action   - - - - Indirect action

When considering breast cancer, one has to bear in mind the sources of these hormones as it is reasonable to expect that many of these tumours will be hormone dependent, although at the present time there is no way of establishing the response of a particular tumour. The largest source of oestrogen and progesterone is found in the ovaries of pre-menopausal women, except during pregnancy. After the menopause, oestrogen and progesterone are secreted in small amounts by the adrenal glands. The anterior pituitary gland is responsible for oestrogen production by secreting adrenocorticosteroid and gonadotrophins, which have a stimulant effect on the ovaries and the adrenal cortex.

The concept of hormonal intervention for breast cancer is not new. The first recorded oophorectomy for this purpose was performed by a Scottish doctor in 1896. Following surgery he found that there was a marked regression of the tumour, and as a result of this, a large trial was conducted in 1900 when regression was noticed in one-third of the patients treated. Following oophorectomy, women will experience the usual menopausal symptoms. It is vital that the patient and her partner are warned of this prior to surgery and symptomatic relief for such symptoms offered postoperatively. The treatment of post-menopausal women and patients relapsing following oophorectomy remained difficult until 1935, when testosterone began to be used in such patients in an attempt to antagonise any remaining oestrogens. The androgens used commonly in treatment now are the drugs Masteril and Durabolin; Durabolin is an oily substance and must be given with a long needle into deep muscle. The side-effects of treatment can be very distressing – the growth of facial hair is particularly worrying to female patients, as the hair is usually dark and quite heavy. Advice concerning its removal may be sought from beauticians; shaving can prove disastrous, but a weekly application of a medically approved hair-removing cream, or facial bleaching, can be useful. The reverse is true on the scalp and thinning is a common occurrence particularly at the temple region. Voice changes can be a permanent effect of androgen therapy, with resultant hoarseness and deepening of the voice. Skin changes are also encountered – an increase in the oiliness of the skin results in open pores and the risk of acne. Strict cleansing of the face should be advised, followed by the use of a good astringent. Greasy food and alcohol should be avoided as they will increase such problems. Increased libido is another side-effect of androgens, but one not often presenting problems. However, patients should be warned of this so that they will at least be prepared and not think that other factors are making them feel more sexually aware.

Along with the development of androgen therapy, surgeons were trying to remove all sources of oestrogens by performing sub-total adrenalectomies; these proved unsuccessful until the advent of oral cortisone preparations in 1950. One year later, a group of patients underwent total bilateral adrenalectomy and favourable results were noted. Prior to performing an adrenalectomy, it is important to explain to the patient that she will need to take oral cortisone for the rest of her life. The side-effects of steroid therapy generally will be discussed later in the chapter.

It seemed probable that the removal of the pituitary gland would have some effect on the progress of the disease, in theory if not in practice. The first hypophysectomy was performed in 1953, with a similar effect to that of adrenalectomy. As the surgical procedure was so daunting, some centres developed a method of ablating the pituitary gland by inserting a radioactive source, usually yttrium, into the pituitary fossa, via the nose. More recent developments in drug therapy, have however, heralded the disappearance of direct attacks upon the pituitary gland.

In the early 1960s, following research into new contraceptive methods as well as work on fertility drugs, the anti-oestrogens were discovered. Subsequently they have been used in the treatment of advanced cases of breast cancer. One of these, tamoxifen, has been found to be very safe and with fewer side-effects, and giving a response in post-menopausal women equally as good as when oestrogens are prescribed.

Two other factors influencing endocrine therapy for breast cancer should be mentioned; the so-called 'disease-free' interval and the menopausal status of the patient. The disease-free interval is the time between initial treatment and the appearance of secondary deposits. If this interval is more than two years, the response to hormonal manipulation is better, although some chemotherapists will argue that if there is a relapse there has never been a disease-free interval. The menopausal status of the patient is particularly important if the patient is less than five years from her last menstrual period. This group of patients are termed perimenopausal and seem to be more sensitive than pre- or post-menopausal women to endocrine therapy.

It must not be forgotten that men may develop tumours of the breast, albeit very rarely; about 3 per cent of all malignancies. A male patient can undergo various hormone manipulations, but hypophysectomy is rarely performed. Seventy per cent will respond to orchidectomy, although this is a short-term measure giving a remission rate of approximately two and a half years.

64 CARE OF PATIENTS ON HORMONAL THERAPY

Oestrogen and progesterone therapy have been found to be of little or no value; corticosteroid therapy can give relief from the pain of bone metastases.

CANCER OF THE PROSTATE

The human prostate is made up of ducts leading to alveoli where the prostate fluid is excreted. The ducts are lined with columnar epithelium rich in calcium citrate and the enzyme acid phosphatase. The secretion of prostatic fluid and the growth of the lining of the ducts are dependent upon the level of circulating androgens. The largest source of androgens is found in the testes, and testicular secretion of androgens is dependent upon the anterior pituitary gland releasing interstitial-cell stimulating hormone. The adrenal glands are also involved because small amounts of androgens are produced in the zona reticulata of the adrenal cortex.

Prostatic cancer is primarily a disease of old age with a peak incidence after the age of sixty. It has been established that nearly all men have hypertrophy of the prostatic gland after the sixth decade. As early as 1616 it was noted by William Harvey that there was atrophy of a bull's prostate following castration. However, this knowledge was not related to treatment until 1930, when an American surgeon named Higgins treated a prostatic cancer by performing orchidectomy on his patients. In comparison to breast tumours, the rationale for hormonal therapy for carcinoma of the prostate is easily understood. The object is to inhibit the production of androgens. While this type of treatment can only be palliative, it can produce an 80 per cent remission rate for approximately two years. The earlier the disease is diagnosed, the more sensitive the tumour will be to endocrine therapy. Unfortunately, because of the often symptomless nature of the disease in its early stages, this advantage cannot always be gained. Patients are usually elderly and the hazards of endocrine therapy have to be weighed against the therapeutic value of treatment. More recently, however, it has been discovered that survival is shorter in oestrogen treated patients than if no treatment is given at all and the only value of oestrogen therapy is for relief of bone metastases.

When patients relapse following successful endocrine therapy, the next stage may be adrenalectomy, or the use of cytotoxic drugs. The use of oestrogens in male patients will have a feminising effect causing loss of libido, impotence, shrinking of the genitalia and gynaecomastia. This can be disturbing for both the patient and his family. Breast enlargement often causes the most anxiety and the patient is best advised to wear loose-fitting clothes or sweaters so that this is not so noticeable. Sexual counselling may be appropriate for the patient and his partner. Progesterones, steroids and anti-tumour drug therapy may also be used in the management of advanced tumours.

CANCER OF THE BODY OF UTERUS

At the beginning of this century it was suggested that there was a probable relationship between hyperplasia of the endometrium and the onset of malignancy in the uterus. From the onset of puberty until the menopause, the normal endometrium is under the control of hormones. During the first half of the menstrual cycle oestrogen causes the endometrium to proliferate; in the middle of the cycle the corpus luteum secretes progesterone, which develops the endometrium into supportive cells. The glandular epithelium begins to secrete glycogen. Adenocarcinoma of the uterine body is a slow growing tumour which produces symptoms at an early stage of its development. The first line treatment of the disease is by radiotherapy and surgery, which gives good survival rates of over 80 per cent at five years.

It was shown in the later 1950s that large doses of oestrogens could produce cystic hyperplasia leading to possible invasive adenocarcinoma in normal women. With the advent of synthetic progesterones it was demonstrated that this hyperplasia could be reversed. It was not until 1960 that the first successful results were shown, of using synthetic progesterones in the treatment of secondary disease. By giving progesterone therapy a remission in 30 to 40 per cent of patients with secondary disease can be brought about. This is due to the effect that progesterone has in maturing the cells of the endometrium which have become malignant following endogenous oestrogen stimulation. Progesterone is an oily substance, and must be given slowly with a long needle into deep muscle. Orally effective compounds, such as hydroxyprogesterone caproate, have recently become available and are used in preference to injection as they are much stronger and more acceptable to the patient. The side-effects of the progestins are few when compared to other endocrine drugs. Nausea and headache are widely reported and backache and hepatotoxicity have been noted. Progesterone therapy certainly has a place in the treatment of advanced disease, although remission rates are higher in the groups of patients who respond well to primary treatment.

ADENOCARCINOMA OF THE KIDNEY

Although not normally regarded as a gland, the kidney is an organ that functions under hormone control, including anti-diuretic hormone from the pituitary gland and cortisone from the adrenal glands. Following experiments with hamsters it was discovered that adenocarcinoma of the kidney could be induced by prolonged oestrogen therapy. A trial led to progesterone administration to patients with metastatic renal carcinoma, and a response rate of 10 per cent was achieved. This may seem low, but anti-tumour chemotherapy has not proved any more successful, despite the fact that 28 of the available drugs have never been tried and so there is no positive 'proof' either way.

CANCER OF THE THYROID

Primary treatment for carcinoma of the thyroid gland is by complete destruction either by radiotherapy, surgery or a combination of both. This results in the patient becoming myxoedematous unless replacement therapy is maintained. It has been found that thyroxine has a therapeutic as well as a physiological effect. By giving rats thyroid stimulating hormone it was found that thyroid carcinoma developed. Following this there had been speculation as to the action of this hormone, especially in papillary carcinomas. When the thyroid is ablated there is a fall in the thyroxine levels which stimulates the secretion of thyroid stimulating hormone (TSH). If any tumour remains, whether primary or secondary, this will be stimulated too. The administration of oral thyroxine will inhibit the production of TSH and therefore remove the stimulation for tumour growth. Follicular carcinoma shows very little response and anaplastic tumours show no response to TSH.

LEUKAEMIA

Addison first noted that lymphoid tissue increased when there was inadequate secretion of adrenal hormones. Later when ACTH was isolated it was found that its administration led to a decrease in lymphoid tissue. In the late 1940s it was introduced for the treatment of lymphatic leukaemias with good results. It is still used for its strong anti-lymphatic action and is one of the most important drugs used in the treatment of leukaemias with the exception of myelogenous leukaemia. Prednisone is the drug of choice for induction of remission in acute lymphoblastic leukaemia and is an alternative to chlorambucil in chronic lymphocytic leukaemia; it is used in combination protocols for the treatment of lymphomas. The effect of treatment is almost certainly cytotoxic and not hormonal.

Hypercalcaemia

One of the complications of advanced malignant disease is hypercalcaemia. It is most commonly found in patients with bone metastases which cause the breakdown of bone, releasing calcium into the bloodstream. Owing to pain the patient is usually immobile and this aggravates the condition and may lead to osteoporosis. Hypercalcaemia may be precipitated by oestrogen and progesterone therapy and is commonly seen in patients with breast cancer. Hypercalcaemia causes atony of gut smooth muscle leading to constipation, nausea and vomiting and later to paralytic ileus. A raised serum calcium inhibits the action of anti-diuretic hormone on the distal tubules and collecting ducts of the kidneys. This produces a diabetes insipidus-like syndrome leading to dehydration due to polyuria and polydipsia. The central nervous system is also affected, initially causing drowsiness, confusion and disorientation. If the patient is left untreated, psychotic changes occur leading to stupor and coma. These are signs that can be observed and must be reported so that treatment can be commenced as soon as possible; it is a complication that is potentially fatal and nurses have a responsibility to recognise the earliest signs and bring them to the attention of the physicians. Primary treatment for hypercalcaemia is by rehydration with a forced sodium diuresis with three litres in 24 hours. Sodium chloride encourages a calcium diuresis. This is usually given as an intravenous infusion as the patient is often nauseated or vomiting. To treat adequately, the tumour growth must be halted by either hormonal manoeuvre or with chemotherapy; corticosteroids are used as it is possible that they have a direct suppressive effect on bone re-absorption. It is claimed that 80 per cent of patients respond to diuresis and steroid therapy alone. More intensive treatment includes low calcium diet, diuretics and the antitumour antibiotic mithramycin.

Anaemia

In cases of advanced cancer, anaemia is a common occurrence, particularly with the lymphomas. The patient produces antibodies which destroy their own red cells. This is called autoimmune haemolytic anaemia. Prednisone has been found to be an effective treatment by depressing the antibody formation and cellular immunity, so inhibiting the destruction of red blood cells.

THE USE OF PREDNISONE

Prednisone causes an increase in circulating neutrophils and therefore of the white cell count. It is believed that prednisone protects the bone marrow reserves rather than increase the actual number of cells. Patients are thought to be more tolerant of higher doses of anti-tumour drugs if prednisone is part of their drug protocol. Prednisone treatment can stimulate appetite, although the extreme can be reached, particularly in children and a strict watch should be kept on their food intake; prednisone can also increase energy and stimulate a feeling of euphoria, which can be useful in the care of the terminally ill; this latter effect cannot be sustained for long periods, and has been called a 'steroid honeymoon' because the sense of euphoria makes the person unaware of the seriousness of the situation.

SUMMARY OF CAUSE AND EFFECT OF HORMONE THERAPY

Treatment by the glucosteroids is included in many protocols for the management of malignant disease. Steroids are an extremely useful tool, but do have many side-effects which can cause distress or even danger to the patient. The nurse can play a major role in the prevention and minimising of complications, as she is in an ideal position to monitor the day-to-day progress of the patient.

It may be useful to list the side-effects into the system they affect. Corticosteroid therapy causes suppression and atrophy of the zona fasciculata of the adrenal cortex and therefore the hypothalmic pituitary system cannot respond in the usual way to stress. The nurse can help by making sure that as many stressful, anxiety provoking situations as possible are avoided. The patient may not be aware of the type of situations that are stressful, so the nurse should discuss this with both the patient and his family.

In an extreme situation, the patient may develop the shock like condition of acute adrenal insufficiency. The symptoms of early acute adrenal insufficiency include fatigue, muscle weakness, joint pain, fever, anorexia, nausea, dizziness and fainting and dyspnoea. If acute adrenal insufficiency occurs, it is a medical emergency necessitating urgent treatment with intravenous hydrocortisone.

The steroids cause redistribution of fat, and the reason for the characteristic moonface, truncal obesity and buffalo hump of

70 CARE OF PATIENTS ON HORMONAL THERAPY

Cushing's syndrome is still not fully understood. Unfortunately, there is little that can be done to help patients with these problems, but the clever use of make-up and hairstyle can be helpful in slimming the face. The buffalo hump can be hidden under a scarf or shawl and male patients can be advised to wear loose fitting jackets or cardigans.

Patients being treated with steroids often complain of increasing weight. This is due to oedema, consequent upon sodium retention and potassium depletion. Although the patient will eat more and deposit fat, diet can help and the patient should be advised to cook without salt and to avoid salty food and drinks, such as cheese and Marmite. The amount of potassium in the diet can be increased by adding citrus fruits, tomatoes and bananas. Lemon juice is particularly good as it is high in potassium and low in sodium. If injectable medications are required, saline diluents should be avoided. Oedema will also make the skin more liable to break down, and bedfast patients should be turned more frequently; mobile patients should be encouraged to move around as much as possible. Blood pressure may rise, especially during the first two weeks of treatment and particularly in patients with existing hypertension or decreased renal function. Regular blood pressure recording should be taken throughout therapy due to the risk of cardiac failure.

Osteoporosis causing pathological fractures is a common occurrence, particularly in post-menopausal women. This is due to the depletion of potassium and the increased output of calcium and phosphorus. A diet that is high in calcium and protein can be encouraged if the condition of the patient permits. It has been shown that calcium leaves the bones faster in an inactive patient, and therefore the patient should be kept as mobile as possible. Safety measures should be discussed with the patient before discharge so that any changes can be made in the house before return.

Patients also have an impaired healing process due to interference with fibroblasts and granulation tissue. Any wound healing is difficult and delayed and patients should be warned that even a small abrasion will bleed profusely and healing will be

CARE OF PATIENTS ON HORMONAL THERAPY

slow. A card should be issued prior to discharge for the patient to carry with him in case of accidents, when appropriate treatment may not be given if this information is withheld.

Gastro-intestinal disturbances can be a problem as corticosteroids increase the production of hydrochloric acid. An antacid may be prescribed in conjunction with the steroid and the use of enteric-coated tablets should be advised. The nurse can also advise the patient to take his medications with a glass of milk or immediately before a meal. Dyspepsia, peptic ulceration and even perforation of the gastro-intestinal tract are complications of treatment and the nurse should be alert for signs of haematemesis or melaena, as these might be the first signs of ulceration. The ulcers are slow to heal due to the anti-inflammatory effect of the steroids.

Steroid-induced diabetes has been reported. The glucose tolerance of the body is increased by gluconeogenesis and insulin antagonism. This results in hyperglycaemia, glycosuria and decreased carbohydrate tolerance. The signs and symptoms are exactly the same as for a diabetic patient and the nurse should be quick to report polyuria and polydypsia; in some cases, routine urine testing might be indicated. Any sign of pruritis vulvae should be reported and strict personal hygiene maintained by the patient. Symptoms can usually be minimised by decreasing the carbohydrate content of the diet, although some physicians prefer not to do this in patients with terminal disease and will prescribe hypoglycaemic agents instead. Steroid-induced diabetes is reversible by stopping treatment.

Steroids also increase the excitability of the central nervous system and cause alterations in the moods of the patient. Some become euphoric, some depressed, others restless or psychotic. Any change must be reported, particularly threats of suicide, which should be taken seriously.

Steroids lower the production of lymphocytes and make the patient more susceptible to infection. The nurse should place the patient in as clean an environment as possible whilst in hospital. Strict aseptic techniques should be employed when attending to any dressings and stringent hand washing between patients is vital. On discharge, the patient should avoid crowds and family and friends with colds or sore throats.

Patients being treated with systemic steroids may have dermal side-effects. Patients bruise easily and this can be counteracted by increasing the vitamin C in the diet. Generally, the skin becomes more friable and great care must be taken to turn bedfast patients frequently to prevent pressure sores.

Some of the side-effects are as dangerous to the patient as his disease and this must be taken into account before deciding on therapy. The nurse has responsibilities to the patient, the physician and herself. She is responsible for giving the drugs and for assessing their effect. She is the planner of nursing care to prevent complications and to minimise side-effects, and she is the teacher to both patient and family. Side-effects cannot be measured by machines, and in monitoring the progress of the patient, the nurse is of paramount importance. She assesses, records and reports to the physician, but in order to do so she must be familiar with the common problems and the measures needed in preventing them.

4. Management of Intravenous Therapy
by MARILYN D. MARKS BA (Hons.), SRN

Iles and Newman (1975) wrote 'the safe administration of intravenous infusion fluids to hospital patients depends on close collaboration between doctors, who initiate therapy, pharmacists, who supply infusions of suitable quality, and nurses, who usually administer fluids to the patients'.

Venepuncture is now one of the most commonly performed procedures in all branches of medical practice. Since the first crude attempts were made, following William Harvey's description of the circulation of the blood in 1628, the techniques of venepuncture and the subsequent administration of intravenous therapy have become increasingly sophisticated. Shortly after Harvey's discovery, the first experiment to utilise this knowledge took place when Christopher Wren and Robert Boyle between them produced a hypodermic needle and successfully injected opium into the vein of a dog. The first intravenous infusion is thought to have occurred in 1832 when Dr Thomas Latta of Edinburgh gave an elderly cholera victim an infusion of water and sodium chloride. Although too rapid an infusion, (six pints in 30 minutes), his revolutionary thought has been refined and adapted to suit many current needs in the expanding fields of medicine. In this century Werner Forssmann established a procedure for cannulation of the great veins and heart. Following the development by Massa at the Mayo Clinic, of the 'Rochester' over-the-needle type of catheter in 1950, the applied technology of medically orientated industry has enabled the confident widespread use of the procedure of intravenous (IV) placement to become established as the accepted norm for both long-term and short-term infusion.

In the currently expanding spheres of cancer treatments, there are several indications for venepuncture and intravenous therapy, both in the diagnosis and treatment of malignant disease.

1. Diagnostic venepuncture. This is to obtain blood samples for laboratory testing, both of a routine nature e.g. to establish the full blood count of a patient prior to the administration of chemotherapy and for more selective investigations e.g. CEA (carcinoembryonic antigen), a marker substance found sometimes present in colorectal carcinoma.

2. *Monitoring.* In addition to simple venepuncture, venous catheterisation plays a vital role in the care of the critically ill when the superficial veins serve as channels for the catheter to reach the vena cava and the right atrium so that haemodynamic changes occurring in or near the heart can be measured (central venous pressure).

3. *Replacement therapy.* Intravenous infusion has almost completely replaced other routes of administration for fluid and electrolyte therapy, as an accurate and quick method of making precise adjustments for disease induced derangement of fluid dynamics. Blood transfusion therapy is increasing in its use, and technical expertise now permits the administration of individual blood components according to the clinical status of the patient.

4. *Maintenance therapy.* The emphasis on intravenous procedures for the increasingly sophisticated maintenance protocols comes from the accessibility of the peripheral veins of the limbs and other areas (such as the scalp of infants) and the ease with which subtle changes in fluid and electrolyte balance may be adjusted. Blood products may be essential in maintaining a stable haematological picture in many of the malignant diseases.

5. *Drug administration.* The provision for a simple and direct route for giving drugs immediately into the circulating bloodstream is regarded as an obligatory safety precaution in anaesthetic and intensive care practice. In cancer treatments, intravenous administration is frequently the route of choice for chemotherapy, when problems of variable absorption render intramuscular or oral routes less reliable.

Equally, in antibiotic therapy, often a more stable serum concentration of the drug can be maintained by continuous infusion or intermittent intravenous administration.

6. *Parenteral feeding.* It is now possible to supply a patient's complete nutritional requirements by the intravenous route. In

cancer care this mode of nutrition can fulfil an important role, particularly in specific instances when there is obstruction of the gastro-intestinal tract; when tube feeding is not advisable either pre- or postoperatively; when a return to a nutritionally adequate diet is delayed or when malabsorption is a complication. Total parenteral nutrition may also be used as an adjunct to chemotherapy or radiotherapy, preventing general debilitation of the patient whilst undergoing treatment, and thus permitting larger doses of drugs or irradiation than would otherwise be advisable. Requirements for fluid, electrolytes, vitamins and minerals will vary according to the individual patient's condition and continual monitoring is therefore essential as the energy and nutrients supplied must take into account abnormal losses as well as predicted requirements.

Certain clinical conditions necessitate the instigation of intravenous therapy. In a state of coma, fluid is necessary to maintain hydration and electrolyte balance; in organ failure (hepatic or renal) careful restriction and calculation of the required fluid volume is needed; in shock, whether due to circulatory collapse, haemorrhage or vascular pooling, the immediate administration of appropriate intravenous therapy may counteract a life threatening situation. With haemopoietic disorders, gastro-intestinal disturbance (vomiting, diarrhoea, obstruction) and conditions leading to salt or protein depletion, replacement and maintenance therapy may provide a crucial element in the patient's treatment.

A major aspect in the medical and surgical management of malignant disease can therefore be provided by intravenous therapy. With the steadily increasing numbers of patients receiving this treatment in the United Kingdom, (in 1976, of the 10 million infusions given, 2,695,000 had additives), it became necessary to rationalise and co-ordinate the policies regarding the administration of all drugs via the intravenous route. In response to this need, the Department of Health and Social Security (DHSS) published a circular HC(76)9, *The Addition of Drugs to Intravenous Infusion Fluids*, which advocated the establishment of a local policy to review current practice in the addition and administration of drugs via intravenous infusion fluids, and making recommendations relating to training of suitably qualified staff for these procedures, who would be aware of the problems and dangers involved.

The Lancet (1976) clearly understood these dangers, 'Care and observation of "drips" is a job for nurses who understand the implications of inattention. It may be cheaper to employ the right staff than to settle an action for negligence.' With developing standards and protocols, intravenous drugs may need to be given every few hours, and doctors may not be readily available so frequently, especially since in some treatment regimes, strict timing is essential. Difficulty can also arise with the comparatively short 'half-life' of some of the drugs in common use and with the increasing numbers of chemotherapy infusions. This has resulted in the formation in some establishments, of 'teams' of nurses capable not only of maintaining infusions and adding drugs to existing intravenous devices, but also of establishing an intravenous pathway for drug or fluid administration; 'In Service' training schemes, as advocated by the HC(76)9 provide the nursing staff with a detailed knowledge of hazards, side-effects and precautions to be taken during drug administration, whether by straight injection, or by infusion. Continuity of service can thus be provided by the nursing profession, after adequate training in pharmacological aspects of their work, in the storage and dilution of fluids and drugs, in the interaction of those agents and in general management of intravenous therapy.

ADMINISTERING INTRAVENOUS THERAPY

1. Intravenous infusions, which include replacement and maintenance therapy of fluids and electrolytes, blood products, and of nutritional necessities (total parenteral feeding). Drugs may be administered via infusions, which may be short-term (less than 12 hours) or long-term (longer than 12 hours). These drugs are given as additives to the infusion fluid and may include several of the chemotherapeutic agents e.g. methotrexate, bleomycin, or more standard replacement drugs such as potassium chloride.

2. 'Stat' injections, or injections to be given once only. Drugs administered in this way include those given by single venepuncture, and those which are additives to an already existing infusion 'line' via the injection site of the giving set, or directly into a cannula or infusion device. Antibiotic therapy is frequently given by nurses in the latter manner and cytotoxic agents may be injected in either way.

THE PREPARATION OF EQUIPMENT AND THE CHOICE OF DEVICE

Several factors must be considered in the selection of the intravenous device. First, the purpose of the venepuncture will govern the choice of device, and the length of time which the pathway needs to be maintained will decide the appropriate piece of equipment. When a blood sample alone is required a syringe and needle technique is generally used; however, when an exceptionally stable intravenous pathway is required, a long catheter may be inserted. The suitability of the patient's peripheral veins and the nature of the intended intravenous procedure, also governs the type of device used; some cannulae permit greater mobility; for some veins a winged infusion set is more suited. Ultimately the choice of device is dependent upon the method of therapy required, allowing for individual patient idiosyncrasies. Therefore, within the field of cancer treatments the following general principles serve as guidelines in the management of intravenous therapy.

(a) If an infusion is to run for only a short time, (a variable time factor, but at the Royal Marsden Hospital the upper limits falls at 12 hours), a winged infusion set is used as it is both convenient and economical. (b) For a chemotherapy infusion intending to continue for any longer than 12 hours; for general replacement or maintenance therapy; or for the transfusion of blood or blood products, a cannula is normally the device to be inserted. (c) For parenteral feeding a large central vein should be used, (peripheral veins have a high incidence of venous thrombosis, because of the osmolarity of solutions used for long-term intravenous nutrition

78 MANAGEMENT OF INTRAVENOUS THERAPY

and should therefore not be used for this purpose), and for the monitoring of the central venous pressure (CVP), a long catheter is inserted. (d) For single intravenous injections, a winged infusion set is used (Fig 4/1), which can either be withdrawn immediately if the therapy is completed, or may be secured and used for

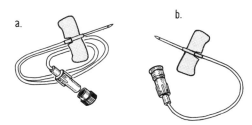

Fig. 4/1 Winged infusion devices with reseal injection site
(a) Winged infusion device   (b) Intermittent winged infusion device

intermittent injections thereafter. If the latter situation exists, a device with a self-sealing injection site can be used, which should be kept heparinised between administrations. If this is not done an accumulation of fibrin will eventually block the lumen of the device.

A similar situation occurs if a cannula is used for long-term administration of antibiotics or cytotoxic therapy, with a Medicut stopper or similar device placed within the lumen (Fig 4/2(3b). This too, will need to be heparinised by the injection of dilute heparin (one part heparin, 1000iu/ml, to nine parts sodium chloride for injection) into the venepuncture device, in a quantity sufficient to displace any medication or blood remaining within the lumen of the tubing or cannula. An alternative to this procedure is the injection of heparin 1000iu/ml directly into the cannula (an amount of approximately 0·2ml, thus filling only the device itself) after adequate flushing of the lumen with normal saline. An obturator (Fig 4/2 (1b and 2b) has been devised, which completely occludes the cannula, projecting a little beyond the tubing into the vein itself, and which abolishes the need for

MANAGEMENT OF INTRAVENOUS THERAPY

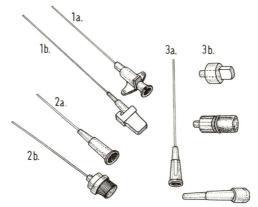

Fig. 4/2 'Needle-through' cannulae, with obturators and stoppers, allowing intermittent administration of fluids (1a) 'Quikcath' (1b) 'Quikcath' obturator (2a) 'Abbocath' (2b) 'Abbocath' obturator (3a) Standard cannula (3b) Plugs on stoppers for adapting standard cannulae for intermittent administration procedures

heparinisation entirely. (This is for use with the Quickcath or Abbocath devices). Should any drug need to be given intermittently into the injection site of an existing intravenous infusion the infusion fluid itself should maintain the patency of the device.

THE DEVICES

The winged infusion set

The winged infusion set consists of a sharp stainless steel needle, two flexible winglike projections mounted on the shank of the needle, a length of flexible tubing and a female Luer adapter which accepts any standard administration set (see Fig. 4/1). Winged infusion sets evolved originally from the scalp vein needle, used for drugs or fluid infusion to infants, when by firm taping of the wings to the flat portions of the head, accidental puncture of the opposite wall of the vein was avoided. The short bevel of the needle and its short overall length also reduces the risk of penetration and allows the nurse or doctor a firm grip and better control during the procedure of venepuncture. Once inserted, the 'wings' may be taped securely into position ensuring the needle will lie safely within the vein. In general, these devices are now regarded as the equipment of choice for percutaneous venepuncture of superficial veins in patients of all ages, preferred for their versatility and ease of manipulation. In straight venepuncture for the collection of blood samples, an ordinary needle and syringe can be used; however the procedure is often less painful using the 'butterfly' type of infusion set and more simply accomplished, particularly if the patient's veins are damaged or relatively inaccessible due to continuous venepuncture and injection of cytotoxic agents. For short-term infusion or intermittent administration of drugs, the lack of bulk in the winged infusion device ensures the minimum of interference in the blood flow past the site of the infusion, thus reducing the risk of local irritation and its sequelae. There is now a wide range of needle sizes which are suited to all routine methods of intravenous therapy.

Indwelling cannulae and catheters

There are three types of indwelling devices used for venepuncture procedures: the plastic-over needle (needle inside) design; the plastic-through needle (needle outside) design; and the plastic or nylon alone (no needle). The insertion of the latter by surgical incision, commonly known as a 'cut down' is now generally reserved for emergencies or surgery to achieve a reliable route for rapid infusion. Percutaneous entry into a vein involves the patient in much less trauma than surgical exposure of the vessel, and there are considerable gains in time and convenience. For many years plastic cannulae were made almost exclusively from polyethylene; nowadays, polyvinyl chloride (PVC), silicone, and Teflon are widely available in different widths (3·30mm–0·45mm) and lengths (1 inch–28 inches), with the advantages of greater flexibility, kink resistance and a reduced chance of thrombo-

MANAGEMENT OF INTRAVENOUS THERAPY 81

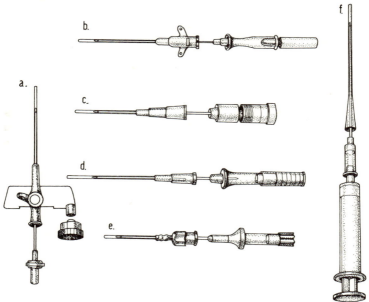

Fig. 4/3 'Needle-through-devices'
(a) 'Venflon'   (b) 'Quikcath'   (c) 'Abbocath–T'   (d) 'Angiocath'
(e) 'Cathlon IV'   (f) 'Medicut'

phlebitis. All varieties of modern cannulae (referring to devices of less than 5 inches in length) resemble each other (Fig. 4/3). There are certain factors which make the choice of device easier, although to some extent this will remain dependent on the personal preferences of the operator.

Ideally the cannulae should be of a one-piece precision moulded design that reduces the risk of breakage under tension and the production of catheter emboli. This avoids the problem of a weak connection between the hub and tube (two-piece design) or of a weakness in the cannula where it is drawn thin to form the relatively large hub (single piece cannula). In the new precision moulded design the cannula is locked into the hub, which itself incorporates a Luer lock for secure attachment of the administration set (Abbocath, Quikath and Angiocath)

Fig. 4/3b.c.d). The cannulae should be radio-opaque to permit them to be visualised during insertion and to allow the localisation of fragments should catheter emboli occur. It is also preferable that the design should allow insertion by no-touch technique and without spillage of blood, while the needle itself should be of a thin wall type to reduce the total bulk and assist simple placement.

The cannula of choice should be the one most suited to the chosen vein; if this is near a joint, a cannula which maintains its patency when kinked is obviously preferred, e.g. Quikcath. In cancer treatments where the veins are frequently used for the administration of vesicant drugs the shorter more flexible cannulae are less traumatic during insertion for the patient and tend to cause less local damage. Some are simpler to use, allowing for single handed removal of the needle if necessary; many have a 'flashback' provision for clear indication of patent vein entry, and wings on some designs allow for ease of taping and manipulation. Despite new and improved devices, some operators persist with the older cannulae, with consequent discomfort and inconvenience to the patient, because of frequent resiting and unnecessary trauma. For specific use where frequent blood samples are required a cannula with three-way tap (e.g. Venflon) may be employed (Fig. 4/3(a)).

Catheters (plastic-through needle type) are devices longer than 5 inches. The general design consists of a sharp hollow needle with a plastic catheter of variable length lying inside its lumen. A stylet, plastic or stainless steel, may be incorporated with these devices, giving rigidity for insertion. The Drum Cartridge Cathe-

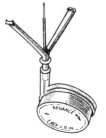

Fig. 4/4 A 'catheter-inside-needle' device wound on a drum

ter gives greater control when placing a long catheter: the stylet and catheter are advanced along the vein through the needle by rotating the drum (Fig. 4/4). Once inserted, correctly positioned, and attached to an infusion, an X-ray will confirm successful catheter placement. For the administration of hypertonic solutions, parenteral nutrition, CVP monitoring, and even occasionally when the patient has no suitable peripheral veins, catheter insertion is an invaluable mode of intravenous infusion.

The choice of giving set

From the steel, rubber and glass assemblies which were in use a relatively short time ago, the development of refined plastic equipment has led to the universal use of prepacked, moulded, one-piece, sterile and disposable units. Pure plastics are seldom used, as the introduction of certain additives produces greater flexibility in a device intended to transfer blood, drugs and parenteral fluids from a container to a patient. PVC is the plastic most commonly used in giving sets. This substance may contain a plasticiser, a stabilising agent, an anti-oxidant and possibly a colouring agent, thus rendering the composition of the tubing as much as 50 per cent of materials other than plastic. 'Leaching' of the constituents of the tubing may cause the transfer of complex and possibly toxic substances into a patient's cardiovascular system or lead to a direct reaction with the electrolytes being infused. Some drugs can be taken up and bound to a plastic complex in a process known as 'adsorption', for example, in an infusion of insulin given to a patient in a diabetic coma via an administration set, as much as 30–40 per cent of the insulin may be removed by the plastic of the set. 'Plastic dust' – minute particles which may inadvertently cause migration of plastic emboli into the arteriovenous networks of the major organs – may induce alterations in liver function tests, or lead to serious problems if the 'dust' should penetrate the brain circulation. Hazards involved in the use of plastics are comparatively minimal when presented against the ease and flexibility, the simplicity of assembly and the disposable nature of the devices.

The introduction of 'inline' filters has been advocated and

several have been marketed which will effectively filter particles at a size ranging from 5 micron (rubber, glass, plastic fragments) to 0·5 micron, (when some bacteria may be trapped). Using such filters there is no clinically significant reduction in the flow rate, except at the smallest diameter. Blood and blood products are obviously unable to be filtered in this way, as the large cells would automatically block the device. This also means it is not possible to use the filters when giving injections directly into a vein, as they would prevent the withdrawal of blood in the syringe in order to buffer the solution injected. The only certain indication for the use of a filtering device is in the injection of intravenous hydroxyurea which is a supersaturated solution, and must not be given if incompletely dissolved. In order to prevent the injection of hazardous particles, by intravenous or intramuscular route, tiny filter aspiration needles can be used to remove particulate matter when aspirating liquid medicaments from glass ampoules, rubber stoppered phials or other containers.

When choosing an administration set, several factors need to be considered. Length and adaptability (with the inclusion of suitable extension sets) contribute towards patient comfort. All sets for blood administration have a drip chamber which has a visible safety filter and which protects against inadvertent transfusion of coagulated matter from blood or blood derivatives. Some chambers are seamless which prevents the accumulation of fibrin and allows the free flow of blood. The second chamber in some administration sets can be used as a pump when pressure transfusion is required, with the floatball occluding the inlet to the upper chamber.

Injection sites in administration sets are an important consideration. Some have 'flashball' sites, with sloping shoulder and injection targets making needle insertion easy, and eliminating the inconvenience of injecting into a small diameter length of rubber tubing. Others incorporate Y-piece injection sites close to the patient, with a leakproof reseal factor. Some sets are made with an integral airway with a non-return ball valve, allowing the addition of drugs by syringe.

Some sets have incorporated airways into their system, others have a separate device for use only with glass bottles. All airways should have a bacteria-retentive air filter, which should always be protected from saturation with infusion fluid. Various types of clamps are in current use. Some involve a secure screw clamp for flow rate adjustment, and slide clamp to interrupt infusion. Others have a 'flo-trol' device allowing for single handed control. One model of this style incorporates a device which enables the administration of fluid to be stopped and restarted without altering the roller adjustment controlling the drip rate.

There are specialised administration sets which are used when extremely accurate measurement of flow rate and precision of volume are necessary. Incorporated into these sets are calibrated 100–150ml chambers, and the drops are produced at a much smaller volume (e.g. 60 drops per ml, whereas normal giving sets deliver fluid at a more standard rate of 15 drops per ml). This factor becomes greatly significant in the delivery of drugs or fluids in paediatric medicine and intensive care. Y-type infusion sets permit either the administration of two fluids simultaneously via one chamber, or via two chambers, meeting only at the cannula connection, allowing for two different rates of infusion via one cannula. If an electronic infusion pump is to be employed to regulate the infusion, it is necessary that the set is a suitable length, and the chambers a correct size to accommodate an electronic drip indicator.

The decision of which administration set to use rests with these factors. All the devices claim to deliver the fluid through a sterile, non-pyogenic pathway; it is the choice of the operator who determines which pathway to be the safest for the patient, and the most convenient for those who maintain the infusion.

Choice of container

No type of container is completely satisfactory in every respect, and care must be taken over some aspects in the use of each kind. There are three main substances of which the containers are made (a) glass, (b) PVC e.g. the Viaflex bag – Travenol, and (c) polyethylene e.g. the Polyfusor – Boots.

(a) The glass container: this always necessitates the use of an airway, but is easy to set up, and the addition and mixing of drugs is simply accomplished. It allows easy examination for particulate content before administration, and the volume of fluid remaining in the container is clearly measurable. Glass bottles are however, heavy and difficult to transport and may contain hairline cracks which allow contamination. These containers are sealed with a rubber bung which may shed rubber particles into the solution, particularly after penetration with an infusion device. Another disadvantage to their use is the possibility of a reaction with the infusion fluid if the contents are alkaline, e.g. sodium bicarbonate. Despite these disadvantages glass containers are often used for the administration of cytotoxic drugs by infusion, e.g. methotrexate, bleomycin, as their suitability exceeds that of the plastic containers, and the possibility of 'leaching' is avoided.

(b) PVC containers: these bags are not fragile and allow for easy examination for contamination. Provided great care is taken over the subsequent mixing it is easy to make drug additions, but constituents of the plastic may contaminate the solution, and adsorption of the drug may occur (see p. 83). No airway is required and the plastic bags can be incinerated; it is difficult to assess the volume of fluid administered. While most hospital staff seem to prefer this container, it is not always possible for it to be used, as the PVC is permeable to water vapour and gases and therefore unsuitable for some solutions e.g. sodium bicarbonate and mannitol. It also provides problems with storage and fluid identification is more difficult due to the translucent outer protective covering.

(c) Polyethylene containers: these containers have the great advantage in that they are suitable for all fluids; the plastic has no additives liable to migrate into the solution, and the walls are not permeable so that solutions like sodium bicarbonate retain their stability. Under normal conditions, these containers have a shelf life of three years. However, it is difficult to examine the container for particles because of its translucency, and again accurate volumes of administered fluids are difficult to assess. In normal use an airway is not required to maintain a closed circuit, but the rate

of infusion may slow as the container collapses, although ultimately it will not allow air to enter the system. The polyethylene container is light, easy to store, and also is the cheapest to stock; it has been found that nurses find it less easy to make drug additions, and to actually set up the infusion.

All the above types of container are likely to remain in general use since hospital produced solutions and preparations for parenteral feeding are often only available in glass bottles, and chemotherapeutic agents are diluted in these containers. However, sodium bicarbonate, phosphates, and from time to time other preparations are only available in Polyfusors, and since most enquiries have shown the PVC bag the easiest for administration and maintenance, it seems clear all three will remain in everyday use.

Choice of solution

Although the choice of infusion fluid rests generally with the doctor and it is his responsibility, (DHSS HC(76)9), to select the correct solution for the clinical status of the patient, it is of great importance that knowledge of the drug reactions that may occur and their cause should be imparted to nursing staff. Most drugs are complex chemicals, and possible interactions are a real hazard in intravenous therapy. Where the management of intravenous fluids and drug additives is the responsibility of the nurse, as happens frequently in cancer treatments, it is important that current knowledge is readily available, and the various principles of drug and fluid interaction are carefully observed.

When one or more drugs are added to an intravenous solution, a reaction may occur which can be observed by a change in the colour of the solution, cloudiness, turbidity or precipitation. These changes may be due to the formation of another chemical; decomposition of the solution; or the production of metabolic substances by the inadvertent introduction of micro-organisms when adding the drug. The fact that no visible change is observed is no guarantee that a reaction has not occurred.

The stability of many drugs is pH dependent. It is essential that

88 MANAGEMENT OF INTRAVENOUS THERAPY

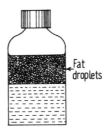

Fig. 4/5 A bottle of intravenous fat emulsion that has 'cracked' after the addition of a drug

a drug which may be alkaline in solution should not be added to an intravenous fluid with an acidic pH, or vice versa. This would hasten the decomposition rate of the additive, and is implicated in the development of hyper-sensitivity. For example, it is unwise to add an alkaline drug such as cephaloridine (Ceporin) to an acidic medium such as Dextrose 5 per cent.

The minute globules of oil or fat which are in suspension to form an emulsion e.g. Intralipid will be 'neutralised' by the addition of a drug, resulting in the separation of the solution into an oily layer and a water layer (Fig. 4/5), and this may produce fat embolism.

Some intravenous fluids are supersaturated e.g. mannitol 20 per cent and sodium bicarbonate, and because of the high percentage of the drug in the solution the addition of another drug may cause a reaction resulting in precipitation. Both these solutions are highly unstable under usual conditions and tend to precipitate normally in glass containers. A solution of mannitol 20 per cent may be re-established by warming the fluid, and may then be utilised in the normal way.

Many drugs react with water and therefore are packed as freeze dried powders and ampoules. The deterioration of the drug in an aqueous solution (hydrolysis) is in most cases quite rapid. If the solution is not used immediately, the drug will be broken down into another chemical or inactivated by the water e.g. penicillin, or mustine (Nitrogen Mustard).

There are a number of factors which may influence these interactions. Drugs in solution are stable for a limited period; therefore it is advisable to mix the drug with the intravenous fluid immediately prior to its use, and to keep the infusion a minimum amount of time. It is usually recommended that bottles of intravenous fluids containing added drugs should be discarded twelve hours after the addition; in many cases, dependent on the solution involved, this limit should be much shorter. The rate at which interaction occurs is influenced by temperature – e.g. a rise of 10 degrees Centigrade will increase the reaction two or three times. It is therefore important that infusions should be kept away from a source of heat.

Some drugs in current use are sensitive to light e.g. amphotericin B (Fungizone), and dacarbazine (DTIC). An infusion of one of these drugs should be covered with black paper to prevent decomposition, and close observation for precipitation is necessary. Likewise some drugs will decompose by interaction with oxygen and carbon dioxide introduced through the airway, e.g. phenytoin sodium, will react with carbon dioxide to give a free base which is insoluble, resulting in a turbidity of the intravenous solution.

A good general rule is that the more complex the solution the more likely it is to break down with the addition of a drug.

A POLICY FOR ADDITION TO INTRAVENOUS FLUIDS

Whenever an addition must be made, adequate information should always be available to the person making the addition. All hospital wards should contain guides to drug incompatabilities which should be continually updated by pharmaceutical staff. As a guideline, the DHSS recommendations are that drugs should never be added to blood products, plasma, fat emulsions, aminoacids, mannitol solutions, Dextrans, sodium bicarbonate solutions, Hartmann's and Ringer's solutions, sorbitol or fructose.

It is considered a wise precaution not to mix drugs unless it is essential and it has been established that they are compatible and safe. This also applies to the mixing of two drugs in a syringe. Many of the problems surrounding the addition of drugs to intravenous fluids could be avoided completely since many potential additives are stable and could be incorporated into the solution during manufacture. One of the commonest additives is potassium chloride, and preparations containing this drug are available commercially. If these solutions were used, the number of drug additions, and hence the potential microbiological hazards would be greatly minimised.

Before the administration of an intravenous drug:

1. The information in the manufacturer's literature should be checked, concerning compatability, and directions for dilution, which will often stipulate the amount of diluent to dissolve the drugs if in a powder form and to which solution the drug should be added. Any queries should be referred to the Pharmacist directly.

2. It is necessary to confirm that the drug is in suitable form for intravenous injection. Some preparations are specifically for intramuscular use only. The pH of the drug and the fluid should be checked for compatability, and the injection prepared.

3. The instructions for mixing and dilution should be followed, taking care to maintain aseptic conditions. If drugs are to be added to an infusion bottle, the solution should be carefully inspected in a good light, for particles and discolouration; the bottle must contain a vacuum, and have no cracks or irregularities since fungal or bacterial contamination can occur. The fluid must be within the expiry date on the label, and the identity of the contents checked.

4. The rubber bung should be cleaned thoroughly using an appropriate disinfectant e.g. 70 per cent isopropyl alcohol, and allowed to dry.

5. Having changed the needle, the drug is injected gently into the bottle, an airway first having been inserted to release the vacuum.

6. It is essential the drug is thoroughly mixed in the fluid, or the patient may be in danger of receiving a concentrated solution. The amount of shaking required to produce a homogenous mixture is generally more than expected, and often it is more difficult to mix solutions in plastic than in glass containers. Incomplete mixing always means that the amount of additive the patient

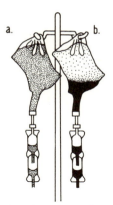

Fig. 4/6 Containers which had had KCl (potassium chloride) added (a) has been mixed (b) has not been mixed

receives will fluctuate throughout the duration of the infusion thus producing a variable response to treatment. The danger involved in the inadequate mixing of an additive can be clearly seen (Fig. 4/6).

7. Labelling and documentation: 'There should be a complete record of all intravenous infusion therapy prescribed for and given to each patient during his stay in hospital. This should include all drugs added to intravenous infusion fluids prior to the commencement of the infusion. It should be on a separate infusion sheet or a separate section of the main prescription sheet and should be retained as part of the patient's permanent medical record.' (DHSS HC (76)9)

The nurse must always chart the infusion of any drug on the appropriate recording sheets, and this should also be included in the Kardex or nursing notes. Bottles and bags containing intravenous additives must have distinctive printed labels attached to the infusion container (Plate 4/1) containing the following information: the name of the patient, the name and dose of the drug added, the date and time of the addition and the name of the nurse responsible.

8. If a reaction occurs during an intravenous infusion, it should be discontinued immediately and the solution replaced with a fluid from another batch number. The pharmacy should be informed of the reaction immediately and all suspect equipment

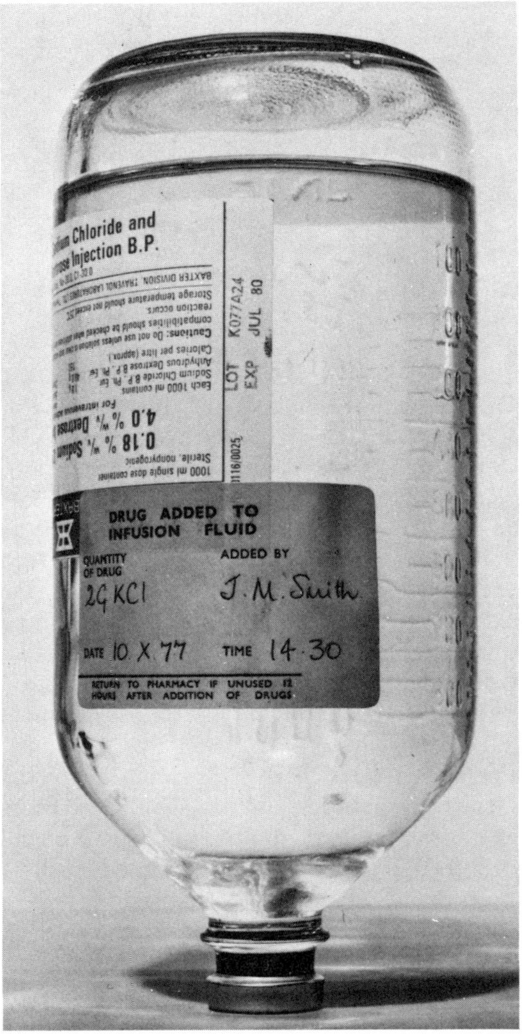

Plate 4/1 Container showing label indicating drug additive to infusion fluid. This indicates patient's name, drug added, time and date of addition and nurse's signature

MANAGEMENT OF INTRAVENOUS THERAPY

retained for inspection. The nature of the defect and time and date of its discovery should be recorded, together with details of the type of fluid, its batch number, expiry date and manufacturer's name.

9. For the direct injection of a drug into an existing infusion, the above method is followed. Once the injection of the drug has been prepared and checked, the patency of the infusion is observed by careful observation of the rate of flow, and the site of cannula entry for any infiltration or phlebitis. After careful cleansing, using a small gauge needle (23G) the drug is slowly injected, with constant inspection of the surrounding tissues for signs of extravasation. The infusion may be stopped during the injection, or if the drug is of a vesicant nature e.g. vincristine, Adriamycin, mustine; some operators will inject the drug into a fast running infusion, in order to prevent scarring of the vein.

The nurse is not expected to know every drug interaction which may occur, but she should have a basic knowledge of the cause of drug and intravenous reactions and be alert to the possibility of their occurrence since she has a great responsibility in the management of intravenous therapy.

PREPARATION OF THE PATIENT

Traditionally, it has always been the role of the doctor to prescribe drugs and the nurse to administer them, so it should follow that the nurse should become skilled and proficient in the administration of intravenous drugs. With this objective, more nurses, particularly in the field of cancer nursing have extended their role to include the placement of intravenous devices for infusion and drug therapy, and therefore, a knowledge of techniques for venepuncture and cannula insertion is becoming increasingly necessary.

In a short visit to the patient before the venepuncture, he/she should be informed and reassured about the procedure. Previous problems with infusions may be discussed and the positioning of the device may be decided, with the use of the non-dominant arm wherever possible. If necessary, because of the administration of cytotoxic agents, an anti-emetic or sedative may be given prior to the venepuncture. The patient should be given the opportunity to visit the bathroom and the environment should be prepared to suit both the comfort of the patient as well as the convenience of the operator, with adequate warmth and lighting. Any long sleeved garment should be removed, at least from the arm to be used.

The preparation of equipment in the clinical room includes the careful priming of the administration set. If a blood transfusion, lipids or protein solution is to be given, the set should be primed with normal saline (0·9 per cent). The procedure of venepuncture should be approached in a calm and positive manner, and comfortable positioning is required both by the person performing the venepuncture and the recipient. A strictly aseptic technique is applied throughout the procedure.

The choice of site is governed by a variety of circumstances and conditions. An unused, easily visible, relatively straight vein away from joints is preferred. There is no one site which is used in every patient, as anatomically and clinically all patients differ. Specific veins utilised for the insertion of cannulae include the cephalic, basilic, and metacarpal veins. For single blood sampling and administering 'stat' doses of drugs intravenously, the antecubital fossa is most convenient, as these veins are usually relatively large and superficial. The age and clinical status of the patient should be considered in the choice of vein, and also the nature of the solution, which may cause much irritation if infused into a small vein (e.g. in parenteral feeding). Contra-indications for the use of a particular vein or arm include sclerosis of the vein, repeated venepuncture at a specific site, scars, eruptions, phlebitis, or lymph node removals during surgical procedures. Tortuous veins, hardened by age or inflamed from previous injections should not be used.

Skin preparation is considered necessary within a hospital (*Drug and Therapeutics Bulletin 1972*) and satisfactory disinfection is achieved with 70 per cent chlorhexidine in spirit or 70 per cent isopropyl alcohol (Mediswab). The site chosen is shaved only if really necessary, for cleanliness and adhesion with tape. The use of local anaesthetic is a much debated issue. Some advocate its use in many circumstances, maintaining the procedure can be extremely painful, but with the new flexible Teflon catheters and skill, the local anaesthetic may cause more discomfort because the patient will feel the first needle entry as well as being aware of vein entry. Occasionally the anaesthetic drug will cause intense stinging and may obscure the vein. In some cases Entonox inhalation analgesia may well remove pain and anxiety from the procedure.

Using strict aseptic techniques the chosen vein is palpated with the tourniquet tightened in position; the patency of the vein is checked by expelling the blood from it and watching it refill. When the area has been thoroughly cleaned (working from the injection site outwards) and is dry, the vein is steadied and the chosen cannula is inserted from above or beside the vein. When evidence of vein entry is obtained by a good flow of blood into the device, the cannula should be advanced in accordance with the manufacturer's instructions. The tourniquet is removed and the giving set connected, and no discomfort should be experienced by the patient and no swelling seen. The device should be taped into position in the way best suited to its design. The tape should not cross the point of entry and should if possible run parallel to the cannula, taping it sufficiently firmly to prevent irritating movement and the transport of cutaneous bacteria into the puncture wound. A safety loop should be made from the giving set and a small dry sterile dressing should cover the point of entry but neither obscuring the cannula tubing nor being totally occlusive, which can increase the underlying cutaneous flora. If a splint is required it should be covered with an absorbent dressing towel to minimise and absorb excessive sweating. A splint is not generally necessary for a cannula inserted anywhere away from a joint, and some of the more flexible and kinkproof cannulae function well, even at an angle in the antecubital fossa, without the need for a splint e.g. Quikcath. The device should be bandaged lightly into place, with a crêpe bandage. The patient should be made comfortable and should be left within easy reach of the nurse call system, his locker and bedtable. The necessary entries on the fluid balance chart, the nursing care plan sheet, and the drug record sheet should be made.

There are certain hazards involved during the actual placement of the device. Particularly there is the possibility of introducing bacterial, viral, protozoal or fungoidal organisms during the procedure through inadequate aseptic technique. There are also non-venous complications of puncture of the vein and subsequent bruising, and extravasation can occur at any stage of the infusion.

Air, particle, or catheter emboli can have serious consequences. Air can be introduced into the system from a badly primed administration set, particles may be infused from anywhere in the administration system – some visible, and many invisible; a catheter embolus may be caused during placement, by the introducer needle being pushed back into the cannula (a procedure which must be avoided) during an attempt at venepuncture; this may sever the end of the cannula, leaving it to enter the circulation, with dangerous consequences.

SUBSEQUENT MANAGEMENT OF INTRAVENOUS THERAPY

Once the intravenous infusion has been established, it is necessary to calculate the rate of infusion and the flow rate. The rate of infusion or drops per minute can be calculated using the following formula

$$\frac{\text{millilitre (ml)}}{\text{hours (hrs)}} \times \frac{15}{60} = \text{drops per minute (dpm)}$$

Key:
millilitre (ml) = number of millilitre in the infusion.
hours (hrs) = number of hours of the infusion.
the multiplication by 15 = number of drops per millilitre in that particular giving set.
the division by 60 is to convert from hours, to drops per minute.
The majority of administration sets in current use have an average of 15 drops per millilitre. Some sets, however, have a smaller microdrip needle for extremely accurate infusion. The drip rate for these is 60 drops per millilitre and the formula would then read:

MANAGEMENT OF INTRAVENOUS THERAPY

$$\frac{\text{ml}}{\text{hrs}} \times \frac{60}{60} = \text{dpm}$$

The rate of flow through an intravenous infusion can vary greatly. The following are some of the factors which may alter the flow rate during administration:

1. The size and choice of device. Changing the radius in the smallest part of the system (usually the needle, cannula or flow control clamp) will alter the flow rate.
2. The construction and management of accompanying equipment.
3. The height of the infusion bottle in relation to the patient.
4. Mechanical properties of the flow control clamp may cause unintentional opening (slipping).
5. Ancillary devices such as filters may obstruct the flow and change the rate.
6. General wear and tear on the plastic tubing by a pinch clamp will change its flexibility.
7. Massed produced administrations sets are generally not precision devices so the size of the drip chamber orifice may be variable.
8. Obstructed vents and airway tubes can inhibit the flow.
9. Clot formation in the lumen of the needle or cannula may slow or stop the flow.
10. An increase in the drop rate results in the formation of larger drops.
11. The viscosity of the intravenous fluid will affect the flow rate. This rate is inversely proportional to the viscosity since it is harder to push fluid through the tubing (rate decreases) as the solution becomes more viscous (viscosity increases).
12. Viscosity is also affected by temperature, e.g. the viscosity of blood increases as the temperature decreases and is about $2\frac{1}{2}$ times greater at 0°C than at 37°C. Blood and water vary to approximately the same extent throughout this temperature range.
13. Patient vascular pressure may alter resistance to the fluid rate.

98 MANAGEMENT OF INTRAVENOUS THERAPY

The use of infusion pumps has facilitated the administration of fluids and drug additives, particularly as timing and volume of the fluid are of great importance in chemotherapy protocols. These machines, e.g. Tekmar T51, have a self-regulating positive pressure action which controls the flow rate despite changes in any of the above mentioned factors influencing flow. The pumps are electrically controlled by a timer (set at the required rate by a digital switch) and a sensor in the photo-sensitive drop detector which registers whenever a fluid drop crosses a light beam. A standard administration set is used and its sterile fluid pathway is not interrupted. The flow rate can be varied (using a 15 drops/ml set) from 4ml per hour to 200ml per hour. In cancer chemotherapy, when high doses of cytotoxic agents are given in an infusion, these pumps act as a regulator and safety precaution. At the Royal Marsden Hospital it has been found that in the administration of high dose methotrexate an infusion pump is of great assistance to regulate the 24 hour infusion (up to 14g has been given by this method). When high dose platinum (up to 200mg) is given, it is accompanied by a forced diuresis necessitating the use of two infusion pumps (connected via a Y giving set to one intravenous cannula); one pump introducing mannitol at a rate of 250ml in 5 hours, the other delivering normal saline 0·9 per cent 1000ml in 5 hours.

THE CARE OF PATIENTS UNDERGOING INTRAVENOUS THERAPY

Any patient, with an infusion in place, whether it be for the administration of a chemotherapeutic drug, for fluid replacement or maintenance therapy will need special care and attention. In some patients this will be limited to care of the infusion and assisting the patient in his necessary loss of mobility and independence, although in some cases of routine therapy the patient may acquire a surprising amount of agility when accompanied by an infusion stand! Others, either due to their clinical status, or as a result of side-effects following drug administration, are in a condition requiring total nursing care in all its diversity. The specific

MANAGEMENT OF INTRAVENOUS THERAPY

management and nursing care of the sequelae of cytotoxic drugs is discussed elsewhere (see p. 38). The importance of asepsis cannot be overstressed, as on every occasion when intravenous therapy is in use, there exists a potential medium for the invasion of micro-organisms. The number of bacteria contaminating intravenous solutions will increase with time and therefore neither bottle nor bag should be in use for longer than 24 hours.

Similarly, administration sets carry the same hazards and Maki (1976) recommends that the entire delivery system down to the cannula (containers and administration sets) be routinely changed every 24–48 hours and at each change of cannula all equipment be totally replaced. Thus it has become policy in many hospitals to change the sets daily and set record labels have been produced to facilitate this aim (Fig. 4/7). These indicate both on the admin-

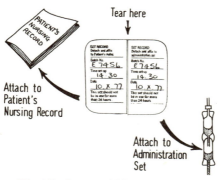

Fig. 4/7 Set record labels showing how information is recorded both in patient's nursing record and administration set

istration set itself, and in the nursing record, when a particular set was first assembled. The set should be changed when the type of solution is changed, e.g. blood to Dextrose solutions and vice versa. Clear fluids, e.g. Dextrose/saline solutions may be administered consecutively via the same system; however the set should always be changed after blood or blood products, lipids or amino-acid infusion.

The dry dressing over the site of venepuncture should be changed daily, following a sterile technique, or more often if this is necessary. If it becomes wet or soiled or needs to be removed for drug administration, a new sterile dressing should be applied. It is advisable to use as little adhesive tape as possible and the use of topical antibiotics is contra-indicated (Iveson-Iveson, 1977). Some operators apply an iodophor spray or ointment, but the efficacy of this practice has not been fully evaluated. Totally occlusive dressings can cause a warm humid environment which encourages the growth of pathogenic organisms. During the changing of the dressing and indeed at any other time if the infusion ceases to function at maximum efficiency, careful inspection of the intravenous site should be made for signs of phlebitis, inflammation, infiltration or purulence. Phlebitis and thrombophlebitis may be caused by chemical irritations of the infused or injected drug, 'leaching' of plastics from the administration system, or occasionally by the invasion of micro-organisms.

Pain, usually one of the first signs of problems with intravenous therapy, occurs at the site of insertion and may extend a variable distance along the vein, accompanied by a redness and slight oedema of the vein itself. The infusion should be resited, or thrombus formation may follow, often accompanied by fever, malaise and leucocytosis. Acute symptoms generally subside in a few days, but tenderness may persist for several weeks. Inflammation is often the precursor to phlebitis or infection, and together with pain and oedema indicates the presence of extravasation (infiltration). In this instance the infusion will have stopped or slowed considerably, and a new intravenous placement will be necessary once these manifestations of infiltration have occurred. Symptoms may be relieved by compresses, e.g. glycerin of icthyol, or chlorhexidine in 70 per cent spirit. It has been recommended that a cannula should be left in place no longer than three days and preferably should be changed every two days (Centre for Disease Control 1973). This principle needs modification when applied to patients receiving frequent chemotherapy, who may have very few available veins, and in this case

MANAGEMENT OF INTRAVENOUS THERAPY

the vigorous adherence to aseptic technique, dressing change and frequent site inspection is most important.

In the daily care of the patient undergoing intravenous therapy, it is the responsibility of the nurse (with regard to accurate monitoring and control of the infusion) to see that protocols are strictly followed; that drugs are given at the correct time; and that adequate records of the drugs, the infusion and fluid intake and output of the patient are correctly charted. The nurse's responsibility also extends to any specific instructions with regard to chemotherapy agents, e.g. to protect Fungizone and DTIC from light during the infusion. As some drugs are unstable in solution, the entire system should be frequently checked for reactions (see p. 87) and care should be taken that the infusion system is not situated near a source of heat, e.g. a radiator, or that a light does not shine on the infusion throughout the night. No infusion should be left in direct sunlight for the same reason.

Intravenous procedures carry certain other hazards for the patient. Apart from complications due to drug, fluid or nutrient infused, venepuncture may have systemic complications resulting from the technique or device used. Septicaemia or bacteraemia has been associated with indwelling intravenous catheters, which should be greatly reduced if meticulous care is taken with aseptic precautions. However, there are numerous potential mechanisms for contamination throughout the infusion device, administration set and container, and each of the twelve connections in the system must be treated with the same rigorous care, for the significance of septicaemia cannot be ignored. The dangers of catheter, particle and air emboli have already been discussed. As with any infusion, the nurse must also be aware of the signs of cardiovascular overloading due to the infusion of too large a quantity or too rapid an infusion. Similarly, the fluid chart may be an early indication of underloading and the development of dehydration or renal failure. With the administration of blood and blood products (particularly white cells and platelets) the nurse must be aware of the signs of a reaction and the importance of crossmatching the correct blood for each individual patient.

102 MANAGEMENT OF INTRAVENOUS THERAPY

SPECIFIC HAZARDS OF INTRAVENOUS THERAPY IN CANCER CHEMOTHERAPY

Infiltration of a cytotoxic agent during administration is a serious complication, owing to the vesicant nature of many of the drugs – the vinca alkaloids, Nitrogen Mustard, Adriamycin, rubidomycin, actinomycin D, Mitomycin C and others. Rapid tissue destruction can occur by extravasation, which may necessitate skin grafting or even amputation. The Editorial of *The Lancet* (1976) stated that most would regard extravasation (tissuing) of an intravenous infusion as no more than a nuisance. Plate 4/2 shows

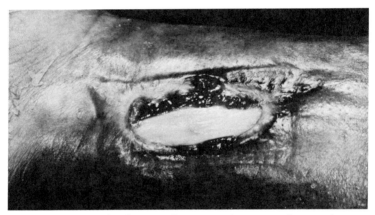

Plate 4/2 Extravasation from a vesicant cytotoxic agent on the ventral aspect of the forearm

an example of such a situation. Once this has occurred the administration should be immediately terminated and an icepack applied. Later, hydrocortisone cream offers some relief and may prevent total destruction.

It is essential to know the drugs which may cause an anaphylactic type of reaction (asparaginase, bleomycin – 3 to 5 hours after administration – and C-Parvum) and to have immediate resuscitation equipment at hand, with hydrocortisone and adrenaline 1:10 000 injections ready. Some drugs are painful when they are given, e.g. DTIC, which causes pain along the vein, and bleomycin which sometimes causes pain in the site of the tumours during administration. Discolouration and scarring of the veins may occur with some of the more vesicant drugs, e.g. Nitrogen Mustard. Instant vomiting occurs when some drugs are administered, probably due to anticipation and psychological response upon seeing the injection, as well as the extreme reactions caused by some of the drugs, e.g. platinum.

SUMMARY

The role of the nurse involved with intravenous therapy carries responsibilities; many of these are encompassed by her traditional caring duties while others are of particular importance in the administration of chemotherapeutic agents via the intravenous route. In all infusion therapy, as cited in HC(76)9 the nurse's responsibilities include:

1. Checking that the container and fluids show no obvious fault or contamination.
2. Checking that the prescribed fluid is administered to the right patient.
3. Observing whether the intravenous line remains patent.
4. Inspecting the site of injection and reporting any abnormality.
5. Controlling the flow at the prescribed rate.
6. Observing and reporting on the condition of the patient, and
7. Maintaining all necessary records.

In cancer nursing, the approach and attitude of the nurse to the patient undergoing cytotoxic therapy is of great significance. There is much she can do to minimise the discomfort and side-effects sometimes experienced (see p. 38) and her awareness and understanding of the therapy can help the patient greatly enhance his own understanding of his condition and treatment. Extending the role of the nurse to include the delivery of intravenous therapy, particularly to patients suffering from malignant disease, can only improve the co-operation between medical, pharmacological and nursing staff, to the amelioration of the physical and mental condition of the patient.

Summary of information relating to the strength, storage, route

Name of Drug (Trade Names)	Average Dose (Approx.)	Strength Available	Storage	Route of Administration
actinomycin D (Lyovac) (Cosmegen) (Dactinomycin)	*Adults:* 0·4mg/m² daily for maximum of 5 days, or *total dose* of 2·4mg/m² over one week *Children:* μgm–0·015mg/kg for a maximum of 5 days	0·5mg 500 micro gms as dry powder vials	Refrigerate	IV
Adriamycin doxorubicin	0·4–0·8mg per kg bodyweight or 60–70mg/m²	10mg 50mg	Room temperature	IV
asparaginase porton	Up to 30 000 units	10 000 units vials 6 000 units vials	Freeze unless otherwise stated by pharmacy	IV
colaspase L asparaginase (Crasnitin)	200 units per kg bodyweight increased to 1 000 units per kg bodyweight	2 000 units 10 000 units vials	Refrigerate unless otherwise stated by pharmacy	IV

dministration, diluents and stability of cytotoxic drugs given parenterally.

iluents	Storage, Stability after Dilution	Other Information
dd 1·1ml water for jection. Add this dextrose 5% lution or sodium loride for an fusion	MUST BE *FRESHLY* PREPARED. DISCARD ANY UNUSED SOLUTION	Give injection directly into the vein or through the tubing of a fast-running IV infusion. *CORROSIVE TO SOFT TISSUE*
mg Dissolved in 5ml ter for injection or rmal saline. *mg* Dissolved in 25ml ter for injection or rmal saline	24 hours at room temperature or 48 hours in refrigerator	Inject through tubing into freely-running IV infusion taking about 2–3 minutes. *AVOID EXTRAVASATION.* Protect from sunlight
issolve dose in 1ml rmal saline then add 9ml	24 hours in refrigerator	Given by doctor because of anaphylaxis
issolve 2 000 unit vial 10ml normal saline. gitate gently to mix	Use within 24 hours Keep in refrigerator	Given by doctor because of anaphylaxis. Slow IV injection or rapid infusion 20–30 minutes in saline. Give test dose intradermally to exclude hypersensitivity

Name of Drug (Trade Names)	Average Dose (Approx.)	Strength Available	Storage	Route of Administration
bleomycin*	5–60mg	15mg amps 5mg amps	Room temperature for 3 years	IM IV IA or local injection into tumour
cytosine arabinoside (Cytosar) (Cytarbarine)	100–200mg or 100mg/m^2	100mg vials	Refrigerate *DO NOT FREEZE*	IV or SC or IT NEVER I
cyclophosphamide (Endoxana)	Up to 1 000–3 000mg/m^2	100mg 200mg 500mg 1g vials	Cool place	IV
dacarbazine (DTIC–DOME)	250mg–400mg/m^2	100mg 200mg vials	Refrigerate	IV
daunorubicin rubidomycin (Cerubidin)	50mg–80mg 0·5–3mg/kg	20mg vials	Room temperature	IV
5-azacytidine	150–400mg/m^2	100mg vials	Refrigerate	IV

Diluents	Storage, Stability after Dilution	Other Information
Normal Saline *IM* Dissolve dose in up to 5ml *IV* Dissolve dose in ml–200ml *Intra-arterial* Make solution 1mg–3mg per ml *Infusion* In saline	Freshly prepared	*IM* Can add 2ml of lignocaine hyd 1% *IV* Inject slowly over a period of 1–2 minutes. *IA* By slow infusion in normal saline *AVOID CONTACT WITH SKIN*
Dissolve contents of vial in 5ml of the special solvent	Store at room temperature and use within 48 hours. Discard any solution which develops a haze	1. Rapid IV injection 2. Infusion over 1, 4, 12 or 24 hours in normal saline or dextrose and saline
Water for injection 100mg in 5ml	Freshly prepared. Stable for 2 hours at room temperature	Direct injection into the vein. *DO NOT MIX WITH ANY OTHER DRUGS* except heparin IA. Infusion recommendations, e.g. 500ml D/S over 1–2 hours
Add 9·9ml water for each injection to each 100mg	Use within 8 hours. Store in refrigerator at 4°C for 72 hours	*AVOID EXTRAVA-SATION* Protect from light. May be given over 1 minute
Dissolve dose in 10–20ml normal saline	Freshly prepared. Store in a refrigerator for 24 hours then discard	Inject into a fast running IV drip infusion. *AVOID EXTRAVA-SATION* Cardiac damage
Add 19·9ml water for injection or normal saline or 5% dextrose. Dilute to 50–200ml	Use within 1 hour	Infuse over 15–20 minutes

Name of Drug (Trade Names)	Average Dose (Approx.)	Strength Available	Storage	Route of Administration
5-fluorouracil	Up to 1g or over for high dose intensive therapy	250mg in 5ml	Room temperature	1. IV infusion 2. IA 3. Oral
azathioprine (Imuran)	Up to 200mg	50mg vial	Refrigerate	Oral IV
melphalan L-phenylalanine mustard (Alkeran)	10mg/day	IV 100mg		Oral IA IV
methotrexate*	1mg–50mg Up to 2g for infusion For intrathecal $12mg/m^2$	5mg in 2ml amps 50mg in 2ml amps	Room temperature	IM IV IT IA
Mitomycin–C	Up to 12mg stat 0·04mg/kg	2mg vial	Room temperature	IP IA IV
nitrogen mustard Mustargen HN2 (mustine)	$6mg/m^2$	10mg vials	Refrigerate	IV IP IA
OIS-platinum diammino chloride	10–50mg (low dose) Up to 200mg for high dose	10mg vials	Refrigerate	IV

Diluents	Storage, Stability after Dilution	Other Information
	Permanent solution	Stat. injection Dilute dose in 500ml dextrose 5%, inject and infuse at rate of 60 drops per minute over 4 hours. Protect from light. Oral preparations available
Add 5ml sterile water/50mg	Use immediately Discard any unused portion	Inject slowly, preferably into tube of running IV infusion. Protect from light. Oral preparations available
10ml own diluent. Mix 1ml of solvent to 100mg. Shake at once, then 9ml diluent added	Use fresh	Inject within 15–30 minutes. Oral preparations available
IT variety in solution	*Normal saline* for IV infusion drip-stable up to 24 hours.	Use *GLASS* bottles. *DO NOT MIX WITH ANY OTHER DRUG.* *Protect from sunlight.*
2mg/5ml dextrose or distilled water	Freshly prepared Store in *DARK* refrigerator if necessary	*AVOID EXTRAVA-SATION.* 10mg dissolved in 500ml 5% dextrose over 1 hour. Protect from light
For IV injection Add 10ml normal saline or water to each 10mg vial	Freshly prepared *immediately* before administration. ($\frac{1}{2}$ life 15 min.)	Inject into tubing of fast-running IV drip infusion
Add 10ml of water for injection to each 10mg	Use within 1 hour. Discard any unused portion.	Follow by normal saline infusion. Special IVI regime for high dose.

Name of Drug (Trade Names)	Average Dose (Approx.)	Strength Available	Storage	Route of Administration
prednisolone sod. phos.	320mg daily	2ml vial	Room temperature	IM IV IA Oral
vinblastine* (Velbe) (Velban)	6mg/m^2 Up to 15mg total dose	10mg vials	Refrigerate	IV
vincristine (Oncovin)	1·4mg/m^2 Up to 2mg maximum dose	1mg vials 5mg vials	Refrigerate	IV

*1. Beware contamination of eyes and skin; goggles and gloves should be worn.
2. After drawing up injections always change needle before administering anti-tumour drugs to patient.

iluents	Storage, Stability after Dilution	Other Information
ready in solution	Use within 24 hours	*IV* Inject slowly over 5 minutes. *Infusion* Add to sodium chloride or 5% dextrose. Use within 24 hours *SENSITIVE TO HEAT* Oral preparations available.
dd 10ml water for jection for each 10mg	In refrigerator 48 hours. If mixed with special diluent in refrigerator for 30 days.	Inject either into vein directly over 1 minute or into tube of fast-running IV infusion. *AVOID EXTRAVASATION.* *WATCH FOR THROMBOPHLEBITIS.*
se own diluent (10ml) add water for injection normal saline, giving oncentration of 01mg/ml to 1mg/ml	Store in a refrigerator up to 14 days	Inject either into vein directly over 1 minute or into tube of fast-running IV infusion. *AVOID EXTRAVASATION.* *WATCH FOR THROMBOPHLEBITIS.* If leakage occurs, apply cold pack.

REFERENCES

Health Services Development Addition of Drugs to Intravenous Fluids, Department of Health and Social Security HC(76)9.

Editorial. (1976). Dangerous Drips. *The Lancet.* i. 291.

Iles, J. E. M. and Newman, M. S. (1975). Infusion Therapy – Problems Encountered by Nurses. *Nursing Times.* 71. 767.

Iveson-Iveson, Joan. (1976). Intravenous Therapy. *Nursing Mirror.* 142. 23.

Maki, D. G. (1976). In *Microbiological Hazards of Infusion Therapy.* Phillips, T., Meets, P., and D'Arcy, P. (Jt. eds.). M.T.P. Press Ltd.

Recommendations for the Prevention of Intravenous associated Infections. (1973). Centre for Disease Control.

The following booklets produced by Drug Companies are very useful – this list is only a selection.

Abbott Hospital Equipment. Abbott Laboratories Ltd., Queenborough, Kent.

Venepuncture and Venous Cannulation. Abbott Laboratories Ltd., Queenborough, Kent.

Information on Intravenous Therapy. Abbott Laboratories Ltd., Queenborough, Kent.

'*Which Intravenous Fluid?*'. Polyfusor, The Boots Company Ltd., Nottingham.

Baxter Administration and Extension Sets. Travenol Laboratories Ltd., Thetford, Norfolk.

A Commitment to Intravenous Therapy. Travenol Laboratories Ltd., Thetford, Norfolk.

The Travenol Guide to Fluid Therapy. Travenol Laboratories Inc. Deenfield, Illinois, U.S.A.

5. Control of Infection in a Cancer Hospital

by EDITH SCOTT SRN, RCNT

The prevention of infection in a cancer hospital is an extension of the basic principles that govern the methods of preventing nosocomial disease in a general hospital. The control of hospital acquired infections depends primarily upon obtaining specific information about the patient and on knowledge of potentially infectious agents and their mode of transmission. The modes of transmission of micro-organisms isolated from cancer patients do not differ from those acquired by other patients. The main concern for the patient with cancer is his lowered resistance to disease caused by these organisms.

Resistance to infection is diminished for two main reasons: first because of the natural history of a particular malignant disease and second, as a result of treatments used to cure or control this disease. It is well established that cancers are more prone to infection than normal tissues. This is brought about by the invasive nature of the disease, eroding blood vessels and causing necrosis often with a super-imposed infection. Neutropenia may occur as a result of invasion of the bone marrow by a primary tumour or secondary deposits. The patient with cancer is often debilitated and in a poor nutritional state; this will affect the skin and mucous membranes, causing loss of continuity and integrity which will permit the entry of endogenous and exogenous microorganisms. Impaired immunological responsiveness may occur in disease processes such as leukaemia and lymphoma.

Treatment aimed at improving the patient's condition may temporarily place him at risk from pathogenic organisms. This may occur when a large volume of tissue is being irradiated and a considerable proportion of the bone marrow is included in the treatment field. Neutropenia may also follow the administration of cytotoxic chemotherapy; this problem is exacerbated when the patient is already neutropenic from his disease, for example, acute myeloid leukaemia. The immunosuppressive action of corticosteroids can bring added risks when used as part of combined therapeutic regimes. The patient is vulnerable not only to recognised pathogens, but also to the normal, localised bacterial flora found within the patient's body, which can cause a generalised infection. The healthy individual is not normally affected by saprophytes in the environment, but these may be pathogenic to the patient with malignant disease (who may become colonised by them).

OPPORTUNISTIC INFECTIONS

These are infections with organisms of low pathogenicity which are harmless to the healthy individual but may infect the highly susceptible patient. A wide range of opportunistic pathogens may be met in the cancer hospital; bacteria, viruses, fungi and parasites.

Bacterial infections

Gram negative low grade pathogens of the klebsiella, pseudomonas and proteus groups, together with saprophytes, may be harboured in moist areas such as around sinks, in floor mops and in nebulisers and humidifiers. For patients with tracheostomies or on assisted ventilation involving nebulisers and humidifiers, particular care and attention is required because of this potential risk. 'Diphtheroids' and coagulase negative staphylococci should not be dismissed as specimen contaminants as these have been known to invade intravenous infusion sites.

Viral infections

Viral infections such as varicella (chickenpox and herpes zoster), herpes simplex and cytomegalovirus are common in phases of inadequate immunological responsiveness. Children with cancer face particular problems from the common childhood infectious diseases.

Chickenpox is a serious hazard to children with acute lymphoblastic leukaemia, both during the initial treatment and also during the period of maintenance chemotherapy. Specific anti-varicella immunoglobulin is available and highly effective if given within 72 hours of exposure. Intravenous cytosine arabinoside or the analogue adenine arabinoside may be given for the treatment of chickenpox. Both these drugs have anti-viral properties although their full potential is not yet known.

Measles is another dangerous infection to a child with acute lymphoblastic leukaemia. Patients who have been in contact with measles and who have not previously been immunised should be given high doses of human immunoglobulin as prophylaxis against the development of giant cell pneumonia and possible central nervous system complications.

Any patient in hospital who requires a transfusion of blood or blood products is exposed to a risk of acquiring hepatitis. The risk is proportional to the amount of blood employed and some blood products such as fibrinogen are more dangerous than whole blood. Any person in hospital who handles blood-contaminated equipment or blood samples, runs a risk of acquiring serum hepatitis. Increased risk of acquiring serum hepatitis is associated with jaundiced patients, patients on immunosuppressive therapy and patients who have had previous blood transfusions. However, it should be borne in mind that in both infectious and serum hepatitis, the virus may be present in blood, faeces, urine and oral secretions. *All* blood should be regarded as hazardous and handled with care.

Fungal infections

Candida infections occur frequently and they are more notable in those patients subjected to multiple and broad spectrum antibiotics or immunosuppressive therapy. Cryptococcal infection is virtually confined to immunosuppressive individuals and should always be considered in the differential diagnosis of aseptic meningitis.

Parasitic infections

Pneumocystis carinii pneumonitis is a much less familiar infection, but is becoming increasingly common in patients with impaired cell-mediated immunity. Little is known of the natural history of the organism, which has the histological appearance of a protozoan. Classically, the patient presents with severe dyspnoea and cyanosis caused by a massive exudate into the alveolar spaces. The lungs are usually the only organs to be affected. It has been found that over 75 per cent of adults have antibodies to pneumocystis in the absence of any history of chest disease. This suggests that many of the infections seen in association with immunosuppression may be reactivation of latent infections which were either mild or sub clinical.

Treatment is usually begun with IM penthadamine isothionate 4mg/kg/day. This has to be continued for 14 days and there is a high incidence of serious toxic effects, mainly renal. Clinical trials with co-trimoxazole in high doses have proved encouraging and side-effects are minimal.

PROTECTION OF THE PATIENT

Bacterial infections are the chief hazard for the neutropenic patient. A wide variety of protective measures have evolved since the concept of reverse barrier nursing was introduced in the early 1960s. The adoption of this principle was in anticipation of the effect on the bone marrow of newly introduced treatments comprising combinations of cytotoxic drugs. These measures necessitate caring for the patient in isolation and at their most stringent entail nursing the patient enclosed in a plastic isolator tent.

Changes in chemotherapeutic regimes have reduced the need for such stringent protective measures except in the case of acute myeloid leukaemia where protective isolation has proved valuable in preventing infections; if patients have marrow transplantation as part of their treatment, protective isolation is essential.

The majority of patients treated today with cytotoxic drugs have only transient neutropenia which can reasonably be

CONTROL OF INFECTION

expected to be measured in days. Where possible, the following precautions should be instigated:

1. The patient should be nursed in a single room.
2. Careful attention be paid to hand washing *before* attending to the patient.
3. Restriction of visitors to relatives and close friends.
4. Exclusion of visitors who have, or who have recently had, infection.

Protecting the neutropenic patient from environmental bacteria still leaves him prey to his own body flora, particularly that of the intestine. To overcome this problem, many centres now use non-absorbable antibiotics given orally to suppress the alimentary flora.

If a generalised infection does occur, successful control depends upon the immediate administration of broad spectrum antibiotics immediately following collection of specimens for bacteriological culture. This is one occasion in which the principle of first isolating the organism and then giving specific treatment should be ignored. A common first choice is a combination of gentamicin and carbenicillin, which can later be modified when the results of the cultures are known.

Knowledge of epidemiological patterns is as important for infection control in cancer patients as it is in other hospital patients. The majority of infections in the cancer patient are caused, however, by micro-organisms coming from endogenous reservoirs such as the oropharynx, gastro-intestinal tract, female genital tract, and the skin. The patient's macrophages may be the reservoir of bacteria and fungi and the cells of nervous tissue reservoirs of the herpes virus. These reservoirs are much more difficult to control. The diagnostic and therapeutic procedures employed in the treatment of cancer may interfere with natural barrier mechanisms and thereby allow either the migration of active micro-organisms or the reactivation of inactive micro-organisms. Exogenous infections play an active role in hospital associated infections affecting the cancer patient. These occur via the usual routes of transmission; contact, ingestion, fomites and airborne. Blood components can be a problem as many patients, especially during chemotherapy and radiotherapy, may require frequent transfusions. There is the additional risk of infection from intravenous sites during chemotherapy and it is important that infusion sets are changed every 24 hours and intravenous devices are changed every 72 hours.

PREVENTION OF INFECTION

The control of nosocomial infections require the following parameters of care:

Formulation of policies and procedures

A Hospital Control of Infection Committee usually formulates policies regarding isolation, use of disinfectants, hospital cleaning, the use of antibiotics and specific aseptic techniques. Admission and isolation policies will indicate the types of infection which should be avoided in an open ward and define which infections require the use of single rooms and the degree of protective measures. Hospital disinfectant policy is essential if they are to be used correctly and in the appropriate concentration. Hospital cleaning procedures should make clear what materials are to be used, the cleaning methods to be employed, the frequency of cleaning required and the storage and maintenance of equipment.

Methods of detecting nosocomial infections

Specific information regarding infections is probably best obtained from the frequent inspection of laboratory reports. This is usually performed on a daily basis by the Bacteriologist and the Infection Control Clinical Nurse Specialist. Each ward is monitored for the type of bacteria present. A card system is often used for each ward and in addition a chart system to give an overall picture. The aim is to be able to pinpoint specific organisms recurring on a ward and to determine the general level of infection. Another method is to report new infections weekly from each ward and to correlate these records with the laboratory results. The records can then be matched against the number of admissions, operations etc., and the rate of infection can be matched with these specific hospital activities.

In most hospitals, there will be many intercurrent infections. Isolation of a strain of bacteria from different sources may be evidence of a cross-infection. If, for example, four cases of an unusually resistant organism were found in one male urology ward during a three week period, environmental swabbing might reveal the organism in the male urinals and also in areas of the sluice. The necessary precautions and procedures against the possibility of further cross-infection might include attention to the bedpan washers or perhaps the introduction of disposable urinals.

Special precautions to eliminate or control sources of infection

This encompasses a wide variety of precautions that will vary according to the type of problem. The action necessary will be decided by the Consultant Bacteriologist, Infection Control Nurse Specialist and other clinical colleagues. A serious problem may involve the Hospital Control of Infection Committee as a whole for decisions. Action may take several lines; noting the type of infection, isolation of a patient, subsequent observation of other patients, barrier nursing, transferring the patient to a special unit, closing and cleaning a ward, etc. In each instance it is essential to weigh the risks of infection against the inconvenience and possible danger, in other ways, of over elaborate measures.

The extent of the problem of nosocomial infection is such that it is advisable for each group of hospitals to have a control of infection nurse in post. She is the key person involved in the investigation of outbreaks of infection and is instrumental in providing the necessary information and action to prevent them. The Infection Control Nurse Specialist plays a vital role in the execution of hospital policies to prevent infection and ensures that procedures and techniques are being performed in the best possible manner.

THE PREVENTIVE ROLE OF THE NURSE

The nurse is in such close proximity with the patient every day of her working life that her role in the prevention of hospital acquired infections is of paramount importance. Prevention is best approached in relation to the three steps by which bacteria bring about infection; that is by consideration of the sources, the routes of spread and the vulnerable sites of infection in the patients.

Sources of infection

The main sources of hospital acquired infections are patients, staff within the hospital and inanimate objects. Nearly all infectious lesions are potential sources but some are more likely to lead to cross-infection than others. Discharging wounds, ulcers, chest infections with heavy expectoration of sputum, infected skin lesions and pressure sores provide a concentrated and constant source of bacteria. Nurses should, therefore, take care when handling these patients or materials that have come into contact with them. A nurse will be in contact with many inanimate sources of bacteria found within the hospital and she must, therefore, be meticulous in personal hygiene and in regular changes of uniform and outdoor clothing.

Routes of infection

The most common route of infection is by the hands. Hand washing must be thorough and in some circumstances an antiseptic preparation is needed. The nurse must also be aware of the other routes of infection; inanimate objects and air currents, other patients, personal visitors and staff who may attend the patient. Cleaning is most important. The use of inappropriate materials and solutions coupled with poor storage practices can result in cleaning being more hazardous than beneficial.

Susceptible patients

Standards of technique should be particularly high in those areas of the hospital where the opportunities of cross-infection are greater. Patients with impaired immunological responsiveness due to natural inheritance, blood dyscrasias, disease processes such as lymphomas and leukaemia and those undergoing therapy with cytotoxic drugs or corticosteroids are particularly at risk. Patients who have been subjected to extensive surgery and those patients suffering from malnutrition and general debility should also be included.

Patients who are at risk from infection may need to be protected by isolation. Where this is not possible or practicable, susceptible patients nursed in an open ward should not be placed in beds close to patients with infections. During venepuncture special care must be taken and the sites of intravenous devices and tracheostomies need special attention; they should be protected from infection by locally applied antiseptics or antibiotics.

Ward staff should record new cases of infection in their wards and be aware of possible relationships to previous infection in other patients. Senior staff should ensure that hospital policies for the prevention of infection are adhered to and help to develop in junior colleagues an appreciation of the hazards of infection in hospitals. Infection control in hospitals is the responsibility of all members of the staff and nurses should become familiar with the modes of transmission of bacteria and possible sources. They should always be on the alert for any breakdown in the methods of prevention of hospital acquired infections.

6. Care of Patients requiring a Pathogen Reduced Environment

by JEAN EDWARDS SRN

One purpose of reverse barrier nursing is to provide a safe environment for the marrow depleted patient prone to infection during or following treatment with combination cytotoxic therapy for different types of malignant disease. This chapter describes a unit mainly concerned with research into, and the treatment of, patients with acute leukaemia and lymphoma. Reverse barrier nursing is also valuable in the early management of aplastic anaemia. Recently with the introduction of bone-marrow transplantation for this disease and also for acute leukaemia, where the patients are deliberately rendered totally neutropenic, 'isolation' and its protective environment is of extreme importance during the recovery period.

The Reverse Barrier Unit at the Royal Marsden Hospital has a complement of sixteen beds, including a six bed open ward used for patients requiring admission for maintenance chemotherapy or blood transfusion. These patients are not neutropenic and therefore no precautionary measures are taken. The remaining ten beds are arranged as two single and four double isolation units, each with its own entry scrub-up area. In the double units, the scrub-up area is situated between the two isolation rooms. Each room has its own shower and toilet. A door leads from the room on to the surrounding balcony and patients may use this facility, providing they avoid physical contact with each other. Another door leads from the corridor and the large window is made of a vibrating plastic, enabling the isolated patient to converse easily with relatives and staff outside the door. Two hatches are set into the corridor wall. The 'clean' hatch incorporates a source of ultraviolet light which kills any surface bacteria. All fresh equipment and articles are passed into the room through

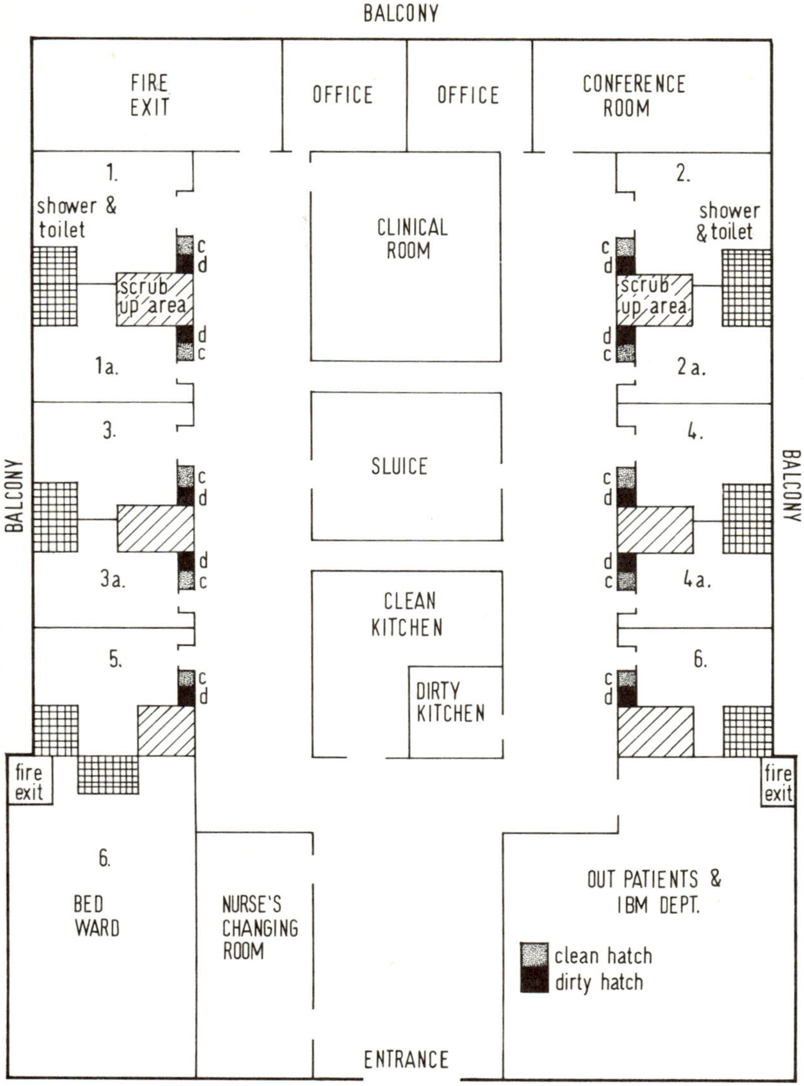

PATIENT CARE IN ISOLATION UNITS 123

Fig. 6/1 Diagrammatic representation of sixteen bed reverse barrier unit

this hatch. All used items from the room are passed back into the corridor via the 'dirty' hatch (Fig. 6/1). The Unit has its own positive pressure air conditioning plant ventilating the isolation rooms, open ward, working areas and the Unit offices. Air is filtered to 0·5 micron to remove dust and bacteria. The temperature is kept constant at 70°F with a humidity of 45 per cent.

To provide a pathogen free environment, meticulous care is given to cleaning within the isolation rooms and includes the use of a 1 per cent solution of a phenolic disinfectant. During patient occupancy all surface areas are cleaned over daily by nursing staff while the domestic staff are responsible for cleaning the shower and toilet areas, the floors and the scrub-up areas. All isolation rooms, the open ward and the working areas are checked weekly by means of settle-plates to ensure that a pathogen free environment is maintained. Between each patient admission, the isolation rooms are carefully cleaned and prepared. Room equipment is removed and sterilised in formalin vapour for twenty-four hours. The furniture is dismantled, turned upside down and the room sprayed using a 1 per cent solution of phenolic disinfectant, then left for at least twelve hours. The room and furniture are then thoroughly cleaned by the domestic staff, after which a nurse dresses as she would if a patient were there and damp-dusts with disinfectant. The furniture is reassembled, the bed made up with clean linen and the room equipment set up, after which the room is again ready for patient occupancy.

All patients admitted to the Unit undergo several routine investigations. A marrow aspirate is taken to establish diagnosis. A full bacteriological screening check is done. Swabs are taken from nose, throat, vagina (female) and any infected lesion. A specimen of stool and a midstream specimen of urine are obtained and sent for culture and sensitivity. The value of screening is to identify the patients' own micro-organisms and later to show 'cross-colonisation' between isolation units. Marker organisms such as pseudomonas and staphylococci can be phagetyped and coliforms with unusual characteristics easily identified. A large volume of blood is taken, some sent for research purposes and the rest for routine investigations, including full blood count, grouping and

X-match, urea and electrolytes, liver function tests, hepatitis-associated antigen (HAA) and coagulation studies. A chest X-ray and electrocardiogram are also performed for diagnostic purposes. Patients have a full nursing assessment and a past medical history taken. They undergo thorough physical examination, special note being taken of areas of sepsis or signs of bleeding.

When the diagnosis is known, both the patients and their relatives are seen and the proposed therapy and its side-effects are explained. Patients with a diagnosis of acute myeloid leukaemia (AML) tend to become neutropenic and prone to infection 3–7 days following therapy with cytotoxic drugs. The isolation regime and the restrictions it imposes are explained to both patients and relatives and their co-operation sought. Relatives and patients are seen separately or together and the intensive nature of the therapy and its possible hazards explained. They are told that there is no cure for this disease, but that if the patient achieves 'haematological remission', the disease can be controlled for a period of time and that when remission is induced and the peripheral blood count is back to normal, the patient will be discharged home. It is stressed that even when in remission, the patient will need to be seen weekly at the hospital as an outpatient and may need admission periodically for blood transfusions and maintenance chemotherapy.

Patients with a diagnosis of AML with a high peripheral white count are put on an IBM cell separator for leucophoresis. This reduces the total white count prior to treatment and the white cells taken off are stored in liquid nitrogen, to be used later for immunotherapy. Patients admitted for marrow transplant undergo the same routine investigations and are transferred into isolation on the day of admission. They are admitted from a waiting list and a full explanation of the procedure and its inherent risks will have already been given both to patients and relatives and a consent form signed. Mothers of children undergoing this procedure are encouraged to stay in the hospital and to dress as the nurses do and go into the isolation room with the child, helping them adapt more easily to the strange environment and routine. Patients with AML can expect to be in isolation for four

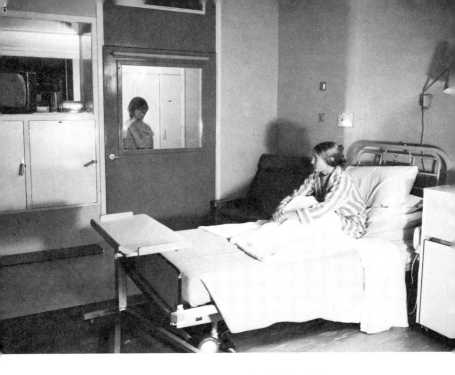

Plate 6/1 The interior of a single isolation room

weeks; patients undergoing marrow transplant for between four to twelve weeks, dependent on whether any complications occur.

Prior to transfer into isolation, patients are bathed and have their hair washed with a preparation containing 20 per cent chlorhexidine gluconate (Hibiscrub). They are wrapped in a sterile sheet and transported to their room, which they enter through the corridor door (Plate 6/1). This door is not opened again until the patient is taken out of isolation.

To prevent the introduction of organisms into isolation, all articles and items of equipment necessary for the care and comfort of the patients are sterilised or disinfected using a variety of methods. Plastic items, e.g. toys, knitting needles and hair rollers are soaked in a solution of 0·5 per cent chlorhexidine in 70 per cent spirit and left for ten minutes. Books, papers, letters, playing

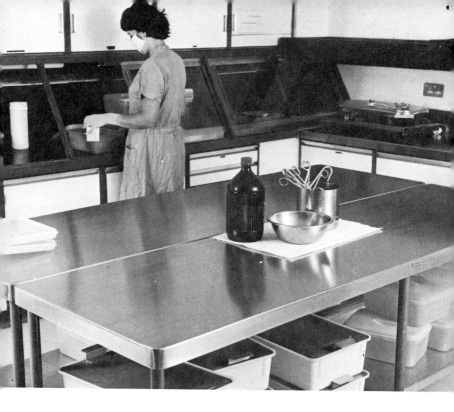

Plate 6/2 The sterile kitchen

cards and cardboard jigsaws are baked in a 'hot air oven' for one hour at a temperature of 150°C. Electrical equipment, e.g. wireless handset, telephone, shavers, calculators, cassette recorders and radios are sterilised in formalin vapour for 24 hours.

There is very close co-operation between the Reverse Barrier Unit and the Central Sterile Supply Department (CSSD). Washbowls, bedpans, urinals, buckets (for cleaning the rooms) as well as the more usual items such as receivers, jugs and gallipots which are made of polypropylene are all sterilised before each use. Bed linen and clothing are usually supplied only freshly-laundered, but in the case of bone-marrow transplant patients, linen also is sterilised. The CSSD may also have to deal with more personal items such as precious cuddly toys or knitting wool. All items are introduced into the room through the clean hatch using a 'no-touch' technique and the ultraviolet light source will kill the few bacteria which may enter accidentally and settle on surfaces.

One of the major sources of infection for the neutropenic patient is from contaminated food. Isolation does impose a few dietary restrictions, but with a relatively small number of patients to cater for, individual preferences can usually be met. All cooking for the isolated patient is done in the Unit's own special kitchen by nursing and ancillary staff trained to the particular requirements of the job by the Unit's Nursing Officer (Plate 6/2). All food is freshly cooked at a high enough temperature and for a sufficient length of time to ensure that all pathogens are killed. Samples of cooked food are cultured by the Bacteriology Department periodically to ensure that standards are being maintained. The greatest risk of contamination is during the serving of food and great care is taken at this point. The serving area is protected by a glass hood and catering staff wear face masks and sterile gloves. All the serving utensils and crockery are washed in a dishwashing machine which rinses at a disinfecting temperature of 90°C for two minutes. They are stored under a glass canopy until used. Food is served using a 'no-touch' technique and carried immediately to the patient in a similarly disinfected container. The lids are removed once inside the hatch and the food taken into the patients' room whilst the containers are left in the hatch, from where they are collected and taken back to the kitchen. All returned items enter the 'dirty' side of the kitchen and only reach the clean side via the dishwasher which is situated in between. All tinned foods and canned drinks are safe to use as they are sterilised during the tinning and canning processes. Dry ingredients such as sugar, tea, salt and pepper are gamma irradiated (by courtesy of the Atomic Energy Establishment) and stored under ultraviolet light as soon as the packets are opened. Butter is melted, reconstituted by beating and stored in the refrigerator until required. Bread is rebaked at 400°F for 25 minutes. Peanuts, crisps and some sweets can be sterilised by baking in the oven for an hour at 400°F. Chocolate can be sterilised by melting it then leaving it to reset under ultraviolet light. Patients' drinking water is sterile and provided by Pharmacy. Its rather flat taste can be disguised by adding tinned fruit juice.

All patients admitted into isolation are routinely started on prophylactic alimentary tract bacterial suppression and antifungal therapy, as it is felt that there is little point in the prevention of acquired infection if the patients are left at risk from their own micro-flora. In a number of centres it has been customary to suppress intestinal flora by non-absorbable antibiotics given by mouth, the most commonly used combination being gentamicin, nystatin and vancomycin. However, it was felt that a combination of framycetin, nystatin and colistin sulphate would be equally effective and cheaper, with less risk of inducing bacterial resistance to valuable therapeutic antibiotics. A two year controlled clinical trial was carried out between both branches of the Royal Marsden Hospital and the Hammersmith Hospital. The preliminary results of this trial have been published and it has been established that patients who receive this prophylaxis have fewer episodes of infection and consequently require less antibiotic treatment. It seems to be of particular value in the prevention of peri-anal sepsis, which is a very serious complication in neutropenic patients and needs treatment which may include temporary colostomy and granulocyte transfusions.

Medical care for the patients is provided from visiting consultants and by a registrar and house physician appointed to the Unit to manage the patients' day to day care. Because of the intensive and detailed nature of the work involved in caring for the neutropenic patient in isolation, a high ratio of nursing staff to patients is necessary. The nursing staff allocation for the Unit is calculated at three nurses per isolated patient in 24 hours. Nursing staff come on duty, change into clean trouser suits and shoes they keep in the Unit. They are given a general ward report before being allocated their patients. Total patient care is practised on the Unit and the nurse is responsible for the day to day nursing management of her patients, including the taking of blood samples for routine examination or for research purposes, the collection of specimens for bacteriological examination and also for the administration of intravenous therapy prescribed, including antibiotic and cytotoxic chemotherapy. The majority of patients have intravenous cannulae in situ for the greater part of their time in isolation and great care has to be taken when dealing with these as the potential risk of introducing infection is so high. Strict aseptic practice is essential.

Before going into the isolation rooms, nurses ensure that all equipment and items necessary for the patients' care have been put into the clean hatch, e.g. bed linen, personal linen, washbowls, dressing packs, bedpans and urinals, etc. Bottles of sterile drinking water and canned drinks are soaked in chlorhexidine solution for ten minutes, then transferred on to the hatch floor, opened and the contents poured into sterile carafes obtained from the clean kitchen. Nurses enter the isolation rooms through the scrub-up areas. They wash their hands and arms up to the elbows, taking care to scrub their nails for five minutes using Hibiscrub. They then don a hat (covering all their hair), face mask and plastic apron and wash their hands again, before entering the isolation room. If one nurse is caring for two isolated patients, the patient with the lowest white count and/or least infection is dealt with first.

Patients shower daily or have a bedbath if unwell, using Hibiscrub. They are examined carefully for signs of bleeding or sepsis, particular attention being paid to the mouth and peri-anal regions, which are common sites of infection in the neutropenic patient. Bacteriological screening is repeated weekly and blood taken twice weekly for full blood count, urea and electrolytes and liver function tests. Full blood counts are taken more frequently if the patients are thrombocytopaenic with evidence of bleeding, e.g. haematuria, bruising or petechial skin haemorrhage. Blood and platelets are ordered as required. Patients having marrow transplants are always transfused with irradiated blood and blood products. Irradiation to 1 500 rads prevents further division of the cells and therefore accidental grafting by stem cells which may be present in the blood. Two-hourly attention is paid to oral hygiene. Following treatment with some cytotoxic protocols, patients may develop severe oral ulceration and are at risk from a superimposed candida infection. For this reason antifungal therapy with amphotericin B lozenges 10mg and nystatin mouthwashes is commenced routinely on admission to the Unit.

Four-hourly observations of temperature, pulse, respiration and blood pressure are recorded. A drop in blood pressure associated with a rise in temperature 12 hours later may be an indication of a Gram-negative septicaemia. Pyrexia in the neutropenic patient is always presumed to be caused by bacterial infection until proved otherwise. Patients with a fever of 38·3°C or more on two consecutive four-hourly recordings undergo the following procedures. They have a thorough physical examination by the Unit's house physician, two separate sets of blood cultures are taken, a midstream specimen of urine is sent for culture and sensitivity and a chest X-ray examination done within 12 hours of the fever. Patients are routinely commenced on IV carbenicillin 5g four-hourly and IV gentamicin, dosage calculated at 5mg per kilogram given in three divided doses over the 24 hour period. This combination of antibiotics is intended to provide broad-spectrum antibacterial cover until an infecting organism is identified, when more appropriate antibiotics may be substituted. If an organism has been cultured, but there is no response to appropriate antibiotic therapy after four days, granulocyte transfusions from a compatible donor will be given.

If no organism is isolated and the fever does not respond, viral studies are performed. Swabs taken from nose, throat and rectum and a specimen of urine are collected into transport medium for virus culture. In addition, viral serological tests are done on paired sera and a blood sample is screened for atypical 'viral' lymphocytes. If the patient has oral candida present and a systemic or oesophageal candidiasis is suspected, anti-fungal therapy with IV amphotericin B may have to be started empirically.

The period of time spent in isolation gives the patients and their relatives the opportunity to know the nursing and medical staff well and the personal relationships formed play an integral part in the patients' care and support. Patients are encouraged to discuss their problems and worries and help is sought from many sources. The Medical Social Worker will help with any social or financial

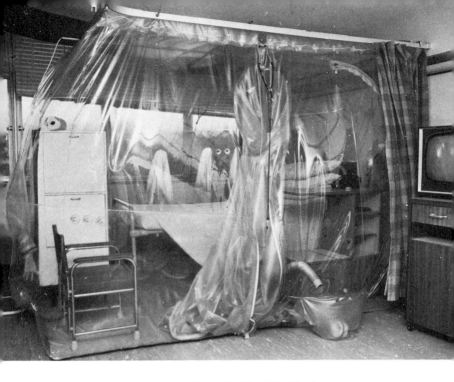

Plate 6/3 The Life Island

problems. Many patients gain great comfort from the regular visits of priests of all denominations. The use of their own telephone helps maintain a link with the world outside hospital and regular visits from friends and family help keep up their general morale. Visiting is allowed at any time and many patients organise a visiting rota of family and friends to cover the whole of the day. Individuals occupy themselves in a variety of ways whilst in isolation. They read, knit, play games or enjoy themselves listening to radio or watching the colour television set provided for each room. Should the patient become seriously ill and not expected to recover, all precautionary measures are discontinued and relatives allowed into the room.

An alternative form of protective isolation is the plastic tent, sometimes called the 'life-island' (see Plate 6/3). One of the major advantages of this type of isolation is that there is a complete physical barrier between the patient and attendants. Nursing and medical staff climb into 'space suits', welded into the isolators' walls, to carry out routine procedures. Procedures are made rather more difficult because of the thickness of the rubber gloves attached to the suit sleeves in comparison with surgical gloves, but with patience, a certain degree of skill is developed. The same supportive measures are required as for the purpose-built unit: adapted air conditioning, sterile food and the co-operation of the CSSD. This type of isolation is suitable for the relatively mobile patient, but not for the seriously ill patient requiring constant attention, or for children. This system of isolation is now used in a number of hospitals where the facilities of a purpose-built Reverse Barrier Unit are not available.

There is still a difference of opinion as to the value of isolation for the neutropenic patient prone to infection, but it seems to be desirable to do what one can within the limits imposed by available resources. It has been demonstrated that isolation prevents the acquisition of organisms from outside and therefore by inference prevents infection.

7. Care of Patients in the Cell Separator Unit

by SUZANNE D. MACKEY SRN

The Cell Separator Unit at the Royal Marsden Hospital is part of the specialised ward that deals with the management of adult acute myeloid leukaemia. This is one of a group of diseases in which cancer develops in the white cell precursors of the bone-marrow, causing a reduction in red cells, white cells and platelets. This is, in turn, associated with anaemia, infection and bleeding and is usually sooner or later fatal. Nevertheless, great advances have been made in recent years in the treatment of acute myeloid leukaemia. This chapter will explain how the IBM Continuous Flow Cell Separator has been involved in these advances and will also discuss its use in other diseases.

PRESENTATION OF ACUTE MYELOID LEUKAEMIA

Patients with leukaemia usually go to their general practitioner because of general malaise, fever, infection or excessive bruising. The general practitioner will arrange for haematological studies which may suggest the possibility of leukaemia, but a bone-marrow aspirate is required to make a definite diagnosis.

PRINCIPLE OF TREATMENT

Because of the seriousness of the disease, patients should be treated as soon as possible. There are two main aspects to treatment of acute myeloid leukaemia. First, an attempt must be made to eradicate all detectable leukaemic cells with chemotherapy. In recent years, several powerful drugs have been developed for this including cytosine arabinoside, daunorubicin and Adriamycin.

PATIENT CARE IN CELL SEPARATOR UNITS

During this period, severe complications including infection and bleeding, can arise and for this reason patients should, where possible, be nursed in reverse barrier conditions. (See chapter 6).

MAINTENANCE TREATMENT IMMUNOTHERAPY

Patients in whom all detectable disease is eradicated with chemotherapy are said to have achieved complete remission (this is now possible in more than 50 per cent of patients). However, it is known that undetectable leukaemic cells persist which eventually cause relapse.

Immunotherapy is a modality of treatment used to maintain the remission of acute leukaemic patients and delay relapse. In man, the first serious attempt at using immunotherapy to treat malignant disease was made by Mathé in Paris. He suggested that in addition to using drugs, it might be possible to stimulate the body's own immune defence mechanisms to find these last few hidden leukaemic cells and kill them. For the treatment of acute myeloid leukaemia at the Royal Marsden Hospital, two types of immunotherapy are used together. The first of these is a vaccine called BCG (Bacillus Calmette-Guérin) which is normally used to prevent tuberculosis. This gives a general boost to the immune system. The second is a preparation of leukaemic cells which experimental evidence has shown to stimulate immunity to this disease, rather like immunisation against infectious diseases (Fig. 7/1). The main purpose of the Blood Cell Separator Unit is to obtain leukaemic cells for immunotherapy using a continuous-flow cell separator and then to administer immunotherapy.

THE IBM CONTINUOUS-FLOW CELL SEPARATOR

The IBM Continuous-Flow Cell Separator is a machine which removes large quantities of white cells or plasma from the blood (see Plate 7/1). This was designed in 1965 by a leukaemia specialist, Dr Freireich, and an IBM engineer. The separator

136 PATIENT CARE IN CELL SEPARATOR UNITS

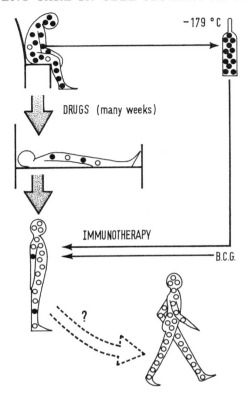

Fig. 7/1 The theory of immunotherapy in the treatment of acute myeloid leukaemia

itself is about the size of a small table which contains a sophisticated centrifuge bowl about the size of a top hat. Heparinised blood from the patient is removed from a vein in the antecubital fossa and pumped into the centrifuge bowl where it is spun and separated into red cells, a buffy layer of white cells and plasma. The buffy coat containing leukaemic cells is removed by a separate pump into a collection bag containing a preservative. Up to 10×10^{12} cells can be collected in a few hours. The gravitational

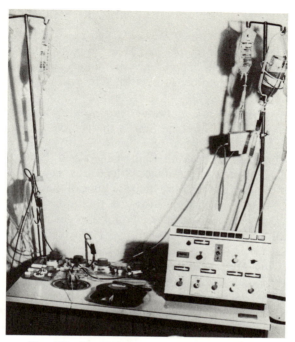

Plate 7/1 The IBM Cell Separator machine in use

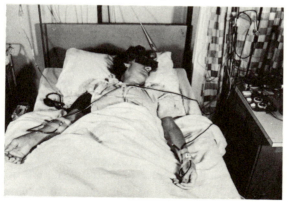

Plate 7/2 A patient attached to Cell Separator machine while in use

force used for separation is low (65G) so most of the platelets remain suspended in the plasma. Meanwhile, peristaltic pumps remove red blood cells and plasma separately from the bowl after which they are recombined and returned into the opposite arm of the donor (see Plate 7/2).

As the separation is a continuous process the volume of blood outside the donor at any one time is the volume in the circuit, approximately 350ml, plus the volume of buffy coat, which is about 400ml in total. All but 40ml of the blood in the circuit is eventually returned to the donor. Blood flow is approximately 40ml per minute, so the entire blood volume of the donor may be processed every two hours. After the procedure, the cells are stored in 2ml glass ampoules over liquid nitrogen at $-179°C$ in a viable condition for immunotherapy. The advantage of being connected to the cell separator machine is that a blood transfusion, which most patients require, can also be given concurrently. Patients with extremely high white cell counts also obtain direct benefit by cell separation which lowers the white cell count. The collected leukaemic cells are concentrated by centrifugation and then sealed in 2ml ampoules for storage in tanks of liquid nitrogen where they can be kept for up to four years. Each ampoule contains approximately 1×10^9 cells. When required, the cells are thawed rapidly at 37°C, washed and resuspended in medium 199 at 4°C and then prepared as a vaccine for immunotherapy.

THE NURSING CARE OF A PATIENT PRIOR TO AND DURING BLOOD CELL SEPARATION

Preparation and care of the equipment

Certain points are of particular importance in setting up the equipment for the cell separator. These concern the protection against the main risks involved in its use which are infection, leakage and air embolus.

PATIENT CARE IN CELL SEPARATOR UNITS

1. Aseptic technique when handling all the equipment is essential. The centrifuge bowl is made of polycarbonate which requires steam under pressure sterilisation (115°C) before each session, but all plastic tubing is pre-packed, sterile and disposable.
2. All tubing and connections must be checked for leakage before starting the procedure and at regular intervals while the patient is on the machine.
3. A bubble detector, which is a small chamber attached to tubing leading back to the donor, will trap any air in the system. This is an extremely important part of the machinery for the nurse to observe. Any sign of air in the chamber (which ought to be detected by an alarm system) means that the inflow to the patient must be clamped off at once with artery forceps.
4. Resuscitation equipment should be readily available and in working order, although providing the above precautions are taken, the risk to the patient is small.
5. Drugs, such as diamorphine, Piriton, hydrocortisone and diazepam may be necessary and should be available.
6. A warm room facilitates the easy flow of blood and it is helpful for the patient if he can enter a warm, bright, cheerful room.

Preparation and care of the patient

On arrival at the Unit, each patient should be assessed individually so that explanations, reassurance and sedation can be given accordingly. A patient who is comfortably settled and who has gained confidence in nursing and medical staff and who understands what is happening to him will be more at ease than one who is left to become uncomfortable and who is frightened and worried. It is helpful to keep certain points in mind.

1. The patient is kept comfortable by supporting the arms on pillows, especially if they need to be kept straight at the elbows, because of the intravenous cannulae. The patient can be helped to sit up or lie back as he wishes and a short sleep will help to pass the time.
2. Explanation and reassurance should be continued throughout the procedure.

3. Appropriate fluids may be given to keep the patient comfortable, but solid food should be withheld as this can induce nausea.
4. It is often helpful for patients' relatives to sit by the bedside; this may help to pass the time more quickly and relieve tension.

Reactions

Sometimes, for reasons not fully understood, patients may have a reaction whilst on the machine. This may present as a rigor or by hypotension with associated faintness, nausea and pallor. These reactions may be due to several factors including anxiety, a transfusion of blood or plasma, or to an excessive rate of blood flow through the machine. A written record giving details of the patients' symptoms is essential if these reactions occur. These reactions are often treated with hydrocortisone, Piriton, Valium and sometimes diamorphine. An important role for the nurse is to be able to recognise warning signs that a reaction is likely to occur: these include listlessness, nausea, yawning, pallor, feeling faint, a feeling of numbness in the fingertips and lips, anxiety and cold extremities.

Special care is needed for a patient who has received intravenous medication while on the machine. His pulse, respiratory rate and blood pressure, colour and general condition should be closely observed and a physician should be present if intravenous Valium (diazepam) is given as there is always a possibility of this causing respiratory depression.

After-care of the patient

Once the intravenous cannulae have been removed, it is very important to make absolutely sure that the veins have stopped bleeding before a dressing is applied. This is vital in patients with low platelet counts. A full blood count can be taken as the cannulae are removed. The patients' temperature, pulse and blood pressure are taken and recorded, together with any special observation which might have been made during the procedure. Patients should be offered refreshments such as coffee and tea at the end of the procedure. When returning to the ward they are

PATIENT CARE IN CELL SEPARATOR UNITS

accompanied by a nurse from the Unit, who gives the ward nurse a full report. Some patients are treated on the cell separator for conditions other than leukaemia and they may go home after the procedure. It is important that these patients are examined by the physician and also given something to eat before leaving.

IMMUNOTHERAPY

As outlined at the beginning of this chapter, the leukaemic cells obtained from the cell separator are eventually used to give immunotherapy to leukaemic patients who have achieved complete clinical remission. These patients are generally well and attend the outpatient clinic of the Cell Separator Unit once a week for their treatment.

Administration of immunotherapy

Immunotherapy is administered by nursing staff. It consists of BCG injected into a limb percutaneously using a Heaf gun which administers 40 needle punctures at a 2mm depth. This gives a dose of approximately 1×10^6 live organisms. At the same time,

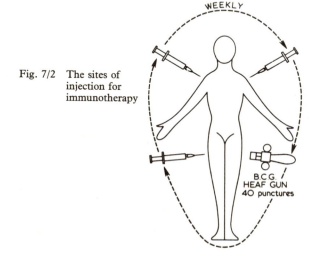

Fig. 7/2 The sites of injection for immunotherapy

reconstituted leukaemic cells are injected intradermally into the other three limbs using a syringe and 21 gauge needle. Approximately 1×10^9 cells are given on each occasion in a total volume of 5ml. (Three limbs are needed because this volume would be too large and painful given in one site alone.) (Fig. 7/2.)

Local reaction to the injection of leukaemic cells is usually limited to transient erythema which disappears within about an hour. The reaction to the BCG is different because it is designed to cause a small crusting lesion about half an inch across which lasts about six weeks. This provides a continuous stimulus to the immune system and in particular the local lymph glands, an important part of the immunotherapy principle. Because of the reaction to BCG a different limb is chosen each week, rotating round all four limbs in turn.

The sociological and psychological aspects of treatment are important because these patients are living from week to week under the threat of a fatal disease. They look upon nursing and medical care with great trust and dependence. The nurses looking after these patients must be sympathetic, have an understanding of the disease and constantly provide reassurance and support. It is important that they realise they have all the time in the world to help these patients who do not.

OTHER USES OF THE CELL SEPARATOR

Granulocyte transfusions

Patients with acute myeloid leukaemia are often very neutropenic, particularly while undergoing intensive chemotherapy and are, therefore, critically at risk to infection. In recent years it has become possible to protect these patients with granulocyte transfusions.

Centrifugal cell separations are not efficient for collecting granulocytes from donors with normal blood counts because the high density of these cells tends to make them sediment in the red cell layer. Therefore a filtration technique has been developed in which the pumps of the IBM machine circulate heparinised blood

PATIENT CARE IN CELL SEPARATOR UNITS 143

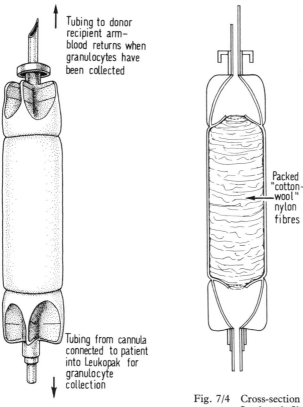

Fig. 7/3 The Leukopak filter

Fig. 7/4 Cross-section of Leukopak filter to show 'cotton wool' nylon fibres

from the donor through nylon fibre columns (Leukopaks) before returning the blood to the donor's other arm (see Figs 7/3 and 4). The granulocytes adhere to the nylon fibres and red cells and plasma return to the donor. The granulocytes are then eluted from the nylon fibres by circulating a litre of ACD (acid citrate dextrose), plasma and saline through each filter. This lowers the pH inside of the filter and causes the granulocytes to detach themselves from the fibres. Up to 6×10^{10} cells can be obtained.

Granulocytes are transfused into the patient after irradiation with 1500 rads to kill donor lymphocytes, thus preventing a serious reaction against the patient called GVH (graft versus host reaction). Irradiation does not affect the granulocytes. The selection of donors is of great importance, as they are giving a service to the hospital as well as to the patient needing granulocyte transfusions. For this reason close family or friends of the patient are desirable, if at all possible, as donors. The nurse will ask the donor to sign a consent form after carefully explaining the procedure and doctors and nurses are always present so that great care of the donor is taken. Interestingly, donors do not get severe reactions as described for acute myeloid leukaemia patients; the only problem may be a vaso-vagal attack during the procedure, which is treated by lying the donor flat, raising the foot of the bed and stopping the machine. As with blood donors, granulocyte donors should be ABO-matched.

Plasma exchange

Certain conditions, and in particular multiple myeloma, are sometimes associated with large amounts of abnormal proteins (paraproteins) in the blood. This condition is called paraproteinaemia. These paraproteins cause an increase in the viscosity of the blood which in turn is associated with clinical problems, including bleeding, cold cyanosed extremities, visual disturbance and neurological abnormalities including profound lethargy and pre-coma. All these clinical signs can be rapidly improved by plasma exchange using the cell separator.

For plasma exchange it is important that the blood is spun at a much higher gravitational force (100G) in the centrifuge than for other conditions described previously. This is so that the patients' platelets are spun free of the plasma and returned to him with the rest of his blood. As the patients' plasma is removed, it is replaced with reconstituted freeze-dried plasma using a dual-channelled pump. About 2–5 litre of whole blood are processed every hour and patients are treated for up to seven hours in a single session without undue discomfort. In addition to paraprotein being removed, other plasma constituents can be collected for estimation and deficiencies in normal immunoglobulins corrected.

Drug overdosage

The cell separator can also be used in the emergency treatment of drug overdosage by removing plasma containing high drug levels and replacing with normal plasma. The principle of plasma exchange described above is the same.

Collection of Rhesus antibody

The principle of plasma exchange can be used to harvest significant amounts of circulating antibody, including for example, Rhesus antibody for obstetrical use.

In the past, the blood cell separator has been used mainly in the treatment of acute leukaemia with immunotherapy. The long-term role of this type of treatment is still being fully assessed. It is very likely that the other uses described in this chapter, including plasma exchange and granulocyte transfusions, will become increasingly important and there seems little doubt that cell separators will benefit both clinical and scientific areas of medicine more and more in the future.

8. The Nursing Management of Children with Cancer

by KATHLEEN PRESTON SRN, RSCN

The prospects for young people suffering from cancer in this country have never been better. There have been steady improvement in treatments and indeed cures are now possible. Nevertheless, there can be no more traumatic experience for a parent than to hear the statement 'your child has cancer'. Almost inevitably this creates a picture of death following a lingering, painful illness. It often means revision of long-term goals for the child with planning on an almost day to day or weekly basis. Once such a diagnosis is confirmed the parents must be told, and at the same time given an explanation of the treatment to be prescribed and the probable course of the illness.

When a child is stricken with cancer the nurse has an unavoidable responsibility for providing emotional support as well as physical care. Furthermore, she must consider the parents and give them such emotional support as they may require; frequently they need more help than the patient. The Platt Committee considered that the sister in charge of a children's ward should be a Registered Sick Children's Nurse, and, there is much to be said for the staff nurses having had similar training.

What attributes should a children's nurse possess? It need hardly be said adequate nursing skills and, in an imperfect world, as many of the human virtues as possible. The latter are almost more important than the former. There must be a genuine love of children and a deep sense of compassion. Emotional maturity or an ability to achieve it is essential, but without becoming hardened. The nurse should possess moral courage, and a gentle sense of humour helps. At all times she must display confidence and be able to give support not only to children but also to their parents. This may appear a formidable list, but it sums up the non-clinical challenge of the problems of children with cancer and the very real and important contribution that nursing staff have to make.

It is arguable that nurses should not spend more than two years in work of this kind. This may be right for some but not necessarily for all. It depends on the psychological compatability of the individual nurse. One should not forget that there is much to be gained from a study in depth of the nursing problems involved; in this context, there can be no better introductory reading for the nurse who may be attracted to this area of work than the proceedings of a conference on the Care of the Child with Cancer held in Washington, U.S.A. in November 1966. The following aspects of the problem were considered:

a. Psychosocial aspects in the care of the child with cancer.
b. Care of the dying child.
c. Care of the family of the child with cancer.
d. Reactions of those who treat children with cancer.
e. Organisational aspects of children's cancer clinics.
f. Role of the nurse in a children's cancer clinic.
g. Role of the social worker in a children's cancer clinic.

Nursing measures employed to maintain optimism and conserve powers of resistance for the child should be flexible, rather than routine. Any therapy, be it surgery, radiotherapy, or chemotherapy, will challenge all the resources that the nurse has at her command. Nursing care is required regardless of prognosis and the nurse must establish good interpersonal relations with both the child and the parents if she hopes to function effectively.

Whilst recognising the value of clinical expertise in paediatric nursing, this must not be at the expense of the child's cultural, social and psychological needs. A child in hospital should never be left alone with his fears and anxieties and the nurse must be alert to recognise changes in the personality of the child as accurately as any physical change in his condition. Whenever possible children should not be placed in a single room; contact with other children makes the adjustment to hospital life more tolerable, although one must always consider the individual child in this respect. Some children, even when quite young, do prefer to have the privacy of their own room. At the Royal Marsden Hospital children are given a choice of accommodation. Neutropenic patients however must, of necessity, be nursed alone. Children with cancer are frequently undernourished as a result of their disease. Ward cooking facilities for use by parents are a great asset, and children will often desire, and eat, food cooked and prepared by their mother. Their individual likes and dislikes can also be catered for. Small, frequent meals high in calorie and protein content should be planned.

AVOIDING INFECTIONS

Perhaps the single most important problem which faces everyone involved in the care of young people with malignant disease is that of infection. Patients with malignant disease have an impaired immunity and an increased disposition to a variety of infections. Whether it is the malignancy which in some way depresses the normal body immune response mechanism, or whether the cancer arises because of the disturbance in the normal immunological response mechanism is not clear. Patients with malignant disease are more prone to infections which afflict the 'normal' population and seem to be more severely affected. Infections with unusual organisms are treated early and vigorously, for what may be a mild infection in a normal child can be fatal in a child being treated for cancer. Fungal and viral infections are especially dangerous.

Whenever possible, exposure to infections must be avoided. Crowded places and indoor parties carry the risk of exposure to coughs, colds and gastroenteritis. For this reason, out-patient clinics should be kept small, approximately eight to ten children if possible. There are obvious advantages in going to school and leading a normal life, but if there is an epidemic of chickenpox or measles it is advisable to keep the child at home and continue studies with the help of a home tutor. Continuing the child's education is very valuable, for learning counteracts boredom and engenders hope. Some risky foods are best avoided, such as 'take-away', spit roast chickens and cold meat pies of doubtful

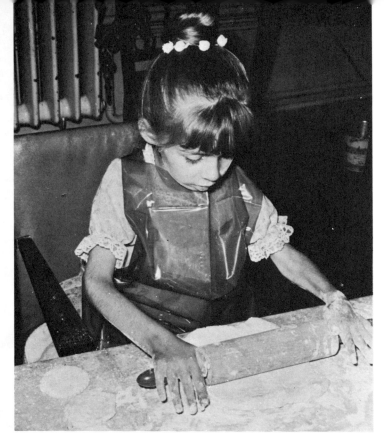

Plate 8/1 Twelve-year-old patient bakes cakes for tea for other children on the ward

age; cream and ice-cream should only be from a reputable source. Foreign travel and food are special hazards.

Certain immunisations and vaccinations should not be given. These include measles, rubella, poliomyelitis and smallpox. Dental care is important, especially for neutropenic patients. Most oncology centres provide a 24-hour telephone service and, if contact with infection does occur, appropriate advice can be given and action taken.

Nursing staff should realise that these children will have periods of remission as well as regression and the nursing care

150 MANAGEMENT OF CHILDREN WITH CANCER

plan needs to take this into consideration. The young patient should be encouraged to function independently. When he is physically able to enjoy play or school work these should be made available, and the help provided by a play therapist is invaluable; children often become very fond of her and gain great comfort and stimulation from her companionship. Frequent outings are to be encouraged when possible and, depending of course on the ages and development of the children, visits to such places as parks, museums, shops, theatres and zoos are stimulating and contribute to good social care (see Plate 8/1). Pets need a mention, for young patients worry considerably about their pets left at home. Nurses should try to remember to enquire after each individual child's pet and, with proper safeguards, even allow pets to be brought to hospital to be seen by the child. If pets are allowed to be kept in hospital, goldfish are about the safest and certainly add a homely touch to any children's ward.

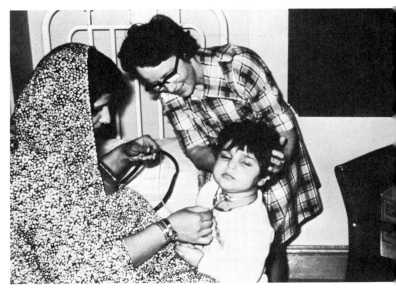

Plate 8/2 Mother of three-year-old Iranian girl being taught to care for the child's permanent tracheostomy. Note that the nurse is in mufti

MANAGEMENT OF CHILDREN WITH CANCER 151

Parents should be allowed to take an active part in the nursing of their child. This contributes to the well-being of the family. It helps parents to feel wanted and useful. If the disease progresses, the nurse should try and ensure that parents do not neglect themselves, particularly in respect of rest and food. The capacity for self-denial which some parents exhibit is amazing, and they need to be encouraged gently, to take care of themselves. Likewise, brothers and sisters should not be forgotten or neglected. Families from other lands present special problems often due to the handicap of language difficulties (see Plate 8/2). Respect must always be paid to their different cultural and social ways of life.

The question of child visitors is often raised. This should be encouraged, certainly in the case of brothers and sisters, provided that the obvious precautions against introducing infectious diseases have been taken. Many of these young patients have to remain in hospital for eight to twelve weeks; this is a long time to be separated from their family and it can be worrying to the children at home.

Unfortunately, owing to the type of therapy which many children have to undergo, many of them will lose their hair (epilation). This can be distressing and careless remarks, although unintentional, can be extremely hurtful. Particular care not to pass such remarks needs to be taken and where necessary visitors should be warned. Wigs are provided for those who desire them.

Many of these patients will be treated with steroids. If side-effects develop such as moonface and growth of facial hair, distress will also be experienced. This is probably more noticeable with girls. These children should be strongly reassured that these effects are not lasting.

An important point is to allow these children to take an active role in their own treatment, and this is helped by giving them simple explanations of their disease and the treatment. These discussions should be appropriate to the age of the child and need not be complete in every detail, but they should help them feel that they can at least partially control the situation. This does sometimes lead to questions – 'Will I grow up?' or 'Will I be cured?'. Whether told directly or not, many of these children know that their disease is life-threatening. This knowledge is created by the necessity for frequent admission to hospital, daily medications, repeated blood transfusions, etc.

THE NURSING CARE OF PATIENTS RECEIVING RADIOTHERAPY

The nursing management of children undergoing radiotherapy is directed towards gaining and keeping their confidence as well as measures to maintain their general well-being and nourishment. The systemic side-effects are not as common as in adults, but when nausea results in refusal to take food and, if vomiting and diarrhoea occur, the significance is greater than in the adult because of rapid dehydration and weight loss. A careful watch must be kept on diet, fluid intake and on body weight; correction of nourishment, fluid intake and electrolyte balance are most important. When radiation induced sickness does occur benefit will be obtained by treatment on similar lines to that given to the adult. In the actual treatment room where they have to be left alone children must be under continual observation through a window or on closed-circuit television. It is often worthwhile having a couple of dummy sessions even if this takes an extra two days, for having once realised that there is no pain associated with the therapy it is remarkable how still they will remain (see Plate 8/3). If sedation is necessary the oral route will be the choice for most children. (At the Royal Marsden Hospital, where possible, radiotherapy is given late in the afternoon so that the child's normal meal times and sleeping pattern are interfered with as little as possible.) Ketalar anaesthesia has its uses but there have been reported instances of bad dreams and nightmares, and very young children cannot tell the nursing staff if they are experiencing such dreams. A period of sleepiness may follow some six to eight weeks after radiotherapy to the head. This usually lasts only a few days, recovery is rapid and complete, but nursing staff need to reassure parents and teenage patients of this possibility.

In view of the possibility of personal exposure to radiation, nurses are required to observe the statutory and hospital Codes of

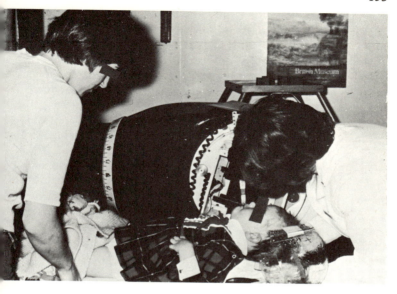

Plate 8/3 Three-year-old child receiving cranial irradiation – note mother helping the therapist

Practice for the protection of persons so exposed. Specialist centres have their own radiation protection service and internal guidance is available.

IMPLANTS AND APPLICATORS

When implants and applicators are used nurses must appreciate the importance of time and distance in relation to radiation. Every nursing procedure which involves close proximity to a patient with a therapeutic amount of caesium or other gamma-emitting radioactive material must be carried out in the shortest time possible compatible with good nursing care. The use of protective lead barriers and trolleys, containers and wall safes will lessen the radiation exposure to all staff in the vicinity. A radiation warning notice must be fixed to the foot of the patient's bed and appropriate nursing instructions placed on the nursing care plan. It is the ward sister's responsibility to organise her staff so that nursing care of the patient is shared and no one will be subject to repeated exposure to radiation. Patients are normally kept in bed during this type of treatment and the bed linen and dressings must be monitored before leaving the ward to ensure that a source has not become displaced. Visitors should be advised to sit several feet from the patient and to keep their visits brief. Children and pregnant women are not allowed to visit the patient during this time.

In the event of death occurring while the radioactive source is still in situ, the nursing staff are responsible for ensuring that the radioactive source is removed before the body is taken from the ward. In the event of any emergency involving radioactive materials, the physics department of the hospital must be informed immediately. Protective clothing in the form of gowns, gloves and instruments must be available for direct handling of patients receiving systemic therapy, such as radioactive iodine.

ANTI-TUMOUR DRUG CARE FOR CHILDREN

Many children are now treated with anti-tumour drugs and the nurse should have a thorough knowledge of the drugs in current use, with particular attention to children's dosage. Parents are, of course, taught by nursing staff how to administer oral chemotherapy at home, side-effects being explained in detail. At the Royal Marsden Hospital a booklet of useful information is given to the parents of children affected by acute lymphoblastic leukaemia, and they are further reassured by the provision of a 24-hour telephone service. Safe custody of drugs taken home is stressed.

PAIN CONTROL FOR CHILDREN

Pain is not the most common accompanying symptom of malignant disease, but when it occurs the harmful effect on mind and body can destroy morale and alter the personality of the sufferer

MANAGEMENT OF CHILDREN WITH CANCER

more effectively than any other single factor. Pain is not always due to the child's cancer, it can be caused by constipation, abscesses, pressure sores, cystitis or anxiety, and these all require appropriate treatment. Young people with cancer can tolerate remarkably high dosage of analgesics; the correct dosage is that which will relieve the pain and not what is thought to be adequate. At the risk of being repetitive let it be said again that most children prefer oral to intramuscular or intravenous medication when possible. A mixture of nepenthe flavoured with blackcurrant syrup is a favourite of the young child, and diamorphine is usually the choice of older children. Pethidine is not reliable when given orally and is of little value in the control of cancer pain. Radiotherapy is often useful in relieving bone pain. Occupational therapy, outings, school lessons, and every possible outlet for relieving boredom will also help to relieve pain.

THE DYING CHILD AND ITS FAMILY

The aim of anyone caring for such a child is not only to help the child but also to help the family accept the loss, which is surely the most profound of all grief. It is as a corporate body that the ward staff should care for such families, and if any member of the ward team has not come to terms with the reality of suffering and death in the world then this is no job for them. Support to the family comes from those who have established the best relations with them. The family will determine this and seek the support for themselves. Great tact and skill is required of hospital staff to encourage parents to give necessary attention to other members of their family. Parents dominated by fear and anxiety for the sick child sometimes hardly realise that siblings are in fact being neglected. All nurses should be constantly on the lookout for such events.

One is rarely asked by a child if he is dying; young children appear to have little concept of dying as a result of illness, they tend to believe that wars, murders and violent crashes are the cause of death; perhaps television has helped to form this view. But there are exceptions and the author has in fact had several teenagers express their fears of dying. Usually it is best to agree that they are very sick but as they have got better on previous occasions hopefully they will do so again. It is perfectly human to say 'I don't know' in answer to some of their questions, which can vary from, 'Nurse, what is it like to die? I don't want to do it, just to know about it, but nobody will tell me'; and further, 'Is heaven nice – but what kind of nice?' Little is gained by being bright and cheerful with the 'everything is going to be fine' approach. Death to most of us is frightening; parents should be allowed to stay with their loved ones, for no one can ever be sure that a dying or apparently dead child does not sense the presence of his parents.

The late Simon Yudkin in *The Lancet* contributed a valuable study in this field which should be read by all engaged in the nursing of children with cancer, 'May I add a plea that we let the dying child die in peace? I am not, of course, referring to an acute crisis in illness which can perhaps be cured but, when the end is inevitable, although we feel the death of a child to be out of time, must we rush around with tubes, injections, masks and respirators? Someone said recently that no-one nowadays is allowed to die without being cured. Perhaps we do it only for the parents' sake; but perhaps we ourselves cannot accept our limitations. And can we sometimes consider whether the dying child should be allowed to die at home? Most parents seem to have accepted what is really a hospital attitude; that death must occur in a hospital – as if to prove that everything has been done. But when the last of the drugs fail in leukaemia or other malignant disease, or where there is chronic progressive cerebral deterioration, should we not at least give the parents the opportunity to choose whether they want their child to die at home rather than in hospital?' There will be few nurses with experience in nursing of children with cancer who would not humbly and respectfully agree.

Following death, the parents should be allowed to express their grief without embarrassment and, if they wish, to help the nurse with Last Offices; The chaplain and medical social worker should be available to offer their skills and practical help if the parents so wish. It is usual to suggest an autopsy, and the parents may well be the first to suggest that this may improve the lot of future patients (provided always that autopsy does not interfere with their religious beliefs). This subject should be brought up for discussion early in the child's illness, and *not* when the child has died.

Experience brings home the fact that more attention should be paid to the needs of parents after their child's death. Many of them have been visiting the hospital for long periods of time, finding there a sense of security and dependence that is difficult to sever when eventually their child dies. They may need advice on how to tell other children about the death of a brother or sister. Members of the nursing staff are often asked to help in funeral arrangements; in choosing between burial and cremation, and so on. Support and advice from the lay administrator are appreciated at this time. Some may think, and rightly so, that these problems are outside the nurse's role, but experience shows that nurses are approached because of the parents' confidence in them, and often there is no one else to turn to. When only one parent is available to cope with this tragedy, the strain is even greater.

The need for support by the people who have shared in the care of the dead child is made obvious by the demand from the bereaved themselves. Many families continue to visit the ward for as long as they feel the need, be it weeks, months or years. On the whole these are not necessarily sad times; it is possible to remember some particularly happy occasion relating to each individual, or to hold small parties for no particular reason except to share in conversation with people whom we have grown quite close to, and with whom we have shared so much. The Society of Compassionate Friends provides comfort and practical help to some of our families.

REFERENCES

Preston, Kathleen (1977). The Nursing Management included in a symposium The Cancers of Childhood. *Nursing Mirror*, **144**, 14.

Yudkin, Simon (1967). Children and Death. *Lancet*, 7 January, 37.

Care of the Child with Cancer. Proceedings of a Conference. *Supp. Journ. Am. Acad. Paed.*, September 1967.

Statistical Report Series No. 2 Report on the Census of Children and Adolescents in non-Psychiatric Wards of National Health Service Hospitals. June 1964 and March 1965. Ministry of Health, HMSO Code 32/528/2/67, page 11, para. 45.

The Welfare of Children in Hospital. Platt Report, October 1958. HMSO Code 32/454, page 10, para. 37.

USEFUL ADDRESS

Society of Compassionate Friends, 8 Westfield Road, Rugby, Warwickshire.

ACKNOWLEDGEMENT

The author is grateful to the Editor of *Nursing Mirror* for permission to reproduce this amended article which first appeared in the *Nursing Mirror*.

9. Nursing Management of the Patient with Pain

by PHILIP HINDS SRN

What is pain? The Oxford Dictionary defines it as 'bodily or mental suffering'. This can only be a simple definition of a complex medical and nursing problem, where diagnosis, measurement and treatment is often at best inadequate and at worst, dangerous.

Pain is a fundamental symptom in medicine and may be regarded as an integral part of human experience. This partly explains why some races or people of differing cultural backgrounds appear to feel less pain than others. Traditionally, warrior races or highly trained soldiers are more stoical; an example being the North American Indian who does not approve of public expression of pain. No definition of pain can ever be satisfactory for it is essentially a subjective phenomenon which only the sufferer can say whether there is pain, where it is and how severe it is. It cannot be shared with anyone and any description will inevitably mean something different to each individual. The word pain has many connotations, from the slang expression a 'pain in the neck' to describe an unwelcome companion, to the severe agony of a broken limb. Apart from the masochist who enjoys pain, most people would agree that pain is an unpleasant sensation to be avoided.

Each person's reaction to pain is complex, for it is influenced by genetics, culture, past experience, emotion, anxiety, religion, the present state of mind and other personal attributes. Any attempt at successful management of pain will need to take these factors into account; a competent nurse should be able to do this. It goes without saying that the prime duty of a nurse is the relief of pain and suffering; she may well be more effective if she has an

160 MANAGEMENT OF THE PATIENT WITH PAIN

understanding of the underlying causation of the sensation which man calls 'pain'.

It is generally agreed that pain is a symptom caused by physical or mental stress and which 'hurts'. It is an unpleasant sensation; it is subjective; it is individual and it is influenced by past experience, emotional states and by degrees of attention. Sternback defines pain as 'whatever the patient says it is and exists whenever he says it does'; this provides a useful premise on which to build a medical or nursing plan of management. Pain may serve either as a warning or as a protection, both in a physical and mental context. As a warning it is one of the symptoms which heralds disease and indicates that examination is necessary to discover the cause. As a protection, such as the pain of an injury which prevents the individual moving and thereby avoids further damage.

The nature of pain is multi-faceted, but some of the basic factors which make up the pain complex include:

Physical and pathological

Bodily pain represents a warning of the danger of harm and is usually considered as having a physical origin which can be isolated to some part of the body. With cancer, there are a number of mechanisms which produce pain that are not always directly due to the actual development of the disease. Mainly, pain occurs when the tumour causes obstruction, but other causes include:

a. compression of nerves by the tumour mass
b. infiltration of nerves and blood vessels by tumour cells
c. ischaemia or distension of abdominal or pelvic organs
d. infection
e. inflammation and necrosis
f. pathological fractures sometimes causing compression of nerves by bone fragments
g. venous thrombosis and pulmonary embolism
h. pressure sores
i. haemorrhoids; constipation and spasms of blood vessels.

Pathological conditions may give rise to pain or may result in

MANAGEMENT OF THE PATIENT WITH PAIN

the patient being more sensitive in his perception of pain and discomfort. Fluid and electrolyte imbalance may result from excessive drainage from fistulae or gastric aspirations, anorexia, vomiting and diarrhoea. These factors are commonly associated with cancer and will inevitably render the patient physically weak, immobile and generally debilitated.

Emotional or psychological

Pain can bring about emotional and psychological changes in even the most well-balanced patient. This can result in the patient becoming withdrawn, sullen, anxious, depressed and even aggressive. The observant nurse will be aware of the patient who has utilised certain psychological defence mechanisms by his regressive behaviour. Such patients will exhibit increased dependency on the staff by constantly seeking care and attention. The nurse will require skill, tolerance and the ability to stand back and observe the situation objectively without personal judgment. Maybe the patient is very frightened for his future or is anxious about his family or mortgage commitments and this is the only way he knows of seeking attention. Equally it must not be forgotten that the quiet patient can also be frightened and worried about his future, but he expresses his suffering in silence; he needs as much care and attention as the attention seeking patient.

Environmental

Environmental factors may contribute to and increase suffering; for example, a noisy atmosphere can prove to be very irritating and further add to the patient's distress. Daytime recreational activities which are not annoying to the patient can help him to forget his pain. With sensible encouragement, the nurse can involve the patient in some of the ward activities, or encourage him to take an interest in his favourite television programme. The occupational therapist can provide diversional therapy and nurses can further help by encouraging friends and relatives to visit, so that pain is no longer a central feature.

Cognitive

This is the significance which the patient places upon his illness, for the nature of illness can influence the individual patient's response to pain. With cancer patients, this is especially so because of the fear and anxiety associated with the disease. The patient may be alarmed and distressed by his condition and this can lead to the pain becoming more intense. Guilt feelings can be an integral feature in the response to cancer and pain. The disease may be regarded as a punishment for something that they have done in the past, and alas, it is commonly believed and supported by the public and many health care professionals alike that cancer patients always experience pain. This is not true; Twycross has reported that as many as 50 per cent of all cancer patients experience no pain or have minimal discomfort, 40 per cent have severe pain and 10 per cent have less intense pain.

The nurse may be able to use a convenient clinical classification to help the medical staff in the management of pain, but all nurses must be on guard since every pain is different and errors of cause may be attributed to this difficulty of differentiation. The nurse must keep an open mind and should not be eager to label patients' pain as psychosomatic or imaginary when there is an absence of conclusive evidence to account for it.

Causes of pain are many and varied and because of this, any attempt at successful management requires thorough assessment before suitable treatment can be initiated.

PAIN RELIEF

The nurse is in a fortunate position within the health care team in that she has more contact with the patient and is available to attend to the patient's needs throughout the day. The nurse's observation of any physical or psychological change and consequent reporting to the doctor will help towards a comprehensive assessment; this in time will be necessary in formulating a suitable medical and nursing plan for a particular patient.

MANAGEMENT OF THE PATIENT WITH PAIN

A number of specialists may be involved in dealing with a patient's pain. This multi-disciplinary approach must be based on consultation and co-operation within a team of experts, which can include surgeon, physician, nurses, psychiatrist, anaesthetist, psychologist, depending on the patient's need and will be supported by physiotherapist, social workers, chaplain, occupational therapist as necessary.

This team approach helps to ensure that the patient is referred to the most appropriate specialist, and thus the most suitable form of treatment for the particular pain can be prescribed. It is the nurse who may be the link in co-ordinating this care.

THE ASSESSMENT OF PAIN

An accurate assessment of pain is necessary for a right diagnosis and treatment. The nursing assessment will take into account the patient's verbal and physical reactions to his pain experience, as well as her own observation. There are three phases of the pain experience; anticipation, presence and aftermath. The nursing assessment is based on the reactions of each phase experienced by the patient. A nursing care history will include the circumstances surrounding the onset of pain, the character of the pain and the site, whether or not it is localised, duration and rhythm and any other related features which will help in forming a pattern which can lead to diagnosis.

The experienced nurse can help the patient discuss his pain so that every aspect is considered. Many patients such as infants, unconscious patients or patients from foreign lands cannot communicate verbally. Some patients find it difficult to describe the pain and its location since there are many descriptions for the sensation, e.g. aching, burning, tingling, sharp, dull, gnawing etc.; these will have different meanings to different people. Where it is possible for the patient to communicate, a more effective and reliable assessment can be obtained. Patients' sound descriptions serve to verify the presence and nature of pain; these can include those sounds which are not true language such as grunting, groaning, screaming, moaning, gasping. These sounds

164 MANAGEMENT OF THE PATIENT WITH PAIN

are involuntary, particularly if pain is sudden, sharp and unexpected and are, therefore, quite an accurate, objective measurement. These sounds can be measured in terms of pitch, volume, frequency and duration. Other reactions which can help to provide a more accurate assessment may take the form of facial expressions and body movements; all these are clues to the presence, severity, duration, location and meaning of pain.

Further assessment of pain may include a physical examination and diagnostic investigations. The nurse's prime concern is to her patient and she will assist in facilitating the investigation by ensuring that the patient does not suffer undue distress. Evidence of suppression or exaggeration of the pain is watched for during the examination. Such non-verbal communications may be accompanied by evidence of autonomic stimulation, e.g. pallor, sweating, dilated pupils, hypertension, tachycardia and increased respirations. The recording of these signs and symptoms will serve as a base line for future reassessment.

MEASUREMENT OF PAIN

There is no reliable method of measuring pain; assessment of pain must be based mainly on the patient's ability and willingness to describe and report his pain accurately.

Where communication is possible and forthcoming, various methods can be employed in an attempt to gauge the degree of pain. One method that can be used by any nurse is to ask the patient to define his pain as mild, moderate, severe or agonising. This can have its problems in deciding how to grade pain when it falls between two categories; a simple variation of this method is the use of the visual analogue scale using a straight line to represent all the degrees of pain between two extremes from 1–10, i.e. 'no pain' to 'intolerable pain' (see Fig. 9/1). The scale can then be measured and the degree of pain expressed as a fraction. This method has been found to have potential for accuracy, providing the patient tells the truth! Similar versions of this method can be used to determine pain relief by comparing the

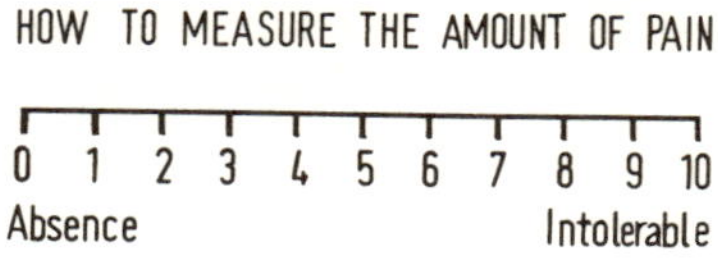

MANAGEMENT OF THE PATIENT WITH PAIN

HOW TO MEASURE THE AMOUNT OF PAIN

```
 0  1  2  3  4  5  6  7  8  9  10
Absence                    Intolerable
```

Fig. 9/1 Diagram showing pain scale measurement

pain before and after treatment using a scale which indicates 'no improvement' to 'complete relief'.

Body diagrams are another simple and useful tool which can be used routinely in the assessment of pain. The patient is asked to locate the site of his pain and this will help the physician and nurse to focus their attention on the cause and thereby contributes to a more accurate assessment.

Individual differences

Only the patient himself knows when the pain, or its effect, is being exaggerated or minimised. To one patient a certain degree of pain will be described as 'severe' and to another 'mild'. Therefore, it must be remembered that it is only the response which can be evaluated and not the pain. Pain intensity is influenced by the patient's own past experience, personality and his present state of mind.

The patient in pain may also have misconceptions about his disease. He may not have been given any information or he may not have understood what he has been told about his illness. By careful listening, the nurse can help to understand and assuage his fears and anxieties as well as helping to clear up misconceptions about the illness, treatment and related factors.

METHODS OF PAIN CONTROL

Advances in medicine have resulted in painful diseases becoming more amenable to treatment. Treatment of pain must be patient-centred and outlined in a plan for each patient. It should be developed by the appropriate team members since there are as

166 MANAGEMENT OF THE PATIENT WITH PAIN

many ways of treating pain as there are causes. Whichever method is adopted to relieve pain will be based on the nature of the pain as well as the expectation of life of the patient. Pain may be acute or chronic.

Acute pain is recognised as short-lived and is amenable to specific measures directed at the removal or healing of affected organs, or on completion of surgical procedures. Chronic pain has probably persisted for a long time and is usually unremitting. The source of such pain may be evident in some cases of inoperable malignant disease and as a guiding rule, symptomatic relief for these patients must be continuous and long-term. Pain may be intractable and not amenable to conventional treatment: in these cases more drastic methods may become necessary such as rhizotomy or chordotomy.

METHODS OF PAIN RELIEF

When the cause of the pain is established, various treatments may be prescribed for its symptomatic relief.

1. Administration of pharmacological agents. These include analgesics, narcotics, tranquillisers, hypnotics, steroids, antibiotics.
2. Interruption of pain pathways:
   a. chemical – nerve blocks using neurolytic agents such as phenol in glycerine which is injected into the intrathecal subarachnoid space thereby destroying specific nerve pathways which transmit pain
   b. electrical (dorsal rhizotomy)
   c. surgical (chordotomy)
3. Electrical percutaneous chordotomy
4. Acupuncture
5. Hypnosis
6. Radiotherapy – especially in the case of metastatic bone deposits
7. Chemotherapy – using cytotoxic agents to inhibit tumour growth

MANAGEMENT OF THE PATIENT WITH PAIN

8. Immobilisation by splinting may be necessary if a pathological fracture is imminent.

If the prognosis is poor, drugs may be used which can have a high incidence of complications, but which are very effective in the short-term. Included in this group are the narcotics, which are of particular use for the patient with terminal cancer and where addiction can be disregarded. When the patient has a normal life expectancy, narcotics should be a last resort, with alternative methods and drugs being first tried to relieve the patient's pain.

It is realised that where a suitable analgesic is chosen and given in adequate dosage, the timing of administration is equally important. In the clinical situation, it is the nurse who administers the prescribed treatment and the time of administration is often left to her discretion. It is essential that the nurse appreciates the principles of drug regimes and their side-effects. Anticipating when the patient is likely to experience pain will be important in successfully spacing treatment and controlling pain.

All drugs should be used at optimum dosage to achieve the desired effect. Dr Cicely Saunders has emphasised the importance of patient participation in deciding what drugs and dosage work best for him, especially in the case of terminal cancer patients. With imaginative and skilful use of drugs, it is rarely necessary to give excessive doses of very potent drugs even in cases of terminal pain. A regular four-hourly interval of administration has been shown to be the regimen of choice for most of the commonly used drugs. The direction *p.r.n.* should be avoided. The nurse must ensure that pain, once abated by regular administration of drugs, does not return. If it does, the patient will lose trust and confidence in the drugs and the competence of the staff and this in turn will lead to fear of further pain and increased anxiety. Fear is a potent antagonist to any drug.

It may be necessary to try various drugs until the best regime is found. The need for pain relief, especially in acute pain, must be balanced against undesirable side-effects which in themselves may be demoralising by rendering the patient drowsy, depressed and totally disinterested in what is going on around him.

168 MANAGEMENT OF THE PATIENT WITH PAIN

The life expectancy of the patient affects the decision to use ablative techniques in the nervous system, not only because of possible complications, but also because the central nervous system can recover. Even when pain pathways in the spinal cord are cut in chordotomy under direct vision, within two to three years a high recurrence rate is experienced.

Apart from the medical management of pain, there are a variety of nursing activities which the nurse can use to assist the patient who is in pain. It is important to realise that pain associated with cancer is often not due to the disease process itself, but may be a nursing problem. Basic nursing procedures must be scrupulously observed – the patient in pain requires skilled and constant nursing care. The nursing intervention is based on the nurses' assessment of the patient and is designed to reduce or eliminate those factors which appear to influence the patient's pain sensation. Nursing activities should be appropriate to the patient's reactions and therefore a patient-centred approach is the surest and most logical method of assistance.

The patient in severe pain is frightened and this fear may arise from various causes. It may be that he is convinced that his pain will continue to get worse or will never be controlled. The nurse can do much to help him overcome his fear by her understanding and sympathetic listening. The nurse must establish a good relationship with the patient and must convey to the patient a genuine desire to help and at the same time the patient needs to be able to trust and to have faith in her integrity. The presence of a nurse with the patient can be therapeutic in itself and physical contact by holding the patient's hand and establishing eye contact can be reassuring for the patient in any phase of pain.

Where applicable, the patient should be fully involved in his own care. Teaching the patient about his pain will include providing as much information as is necessary regarding the nature of the pain, the length of time the pain is likely to last, the quality of the pain sensation and by clarifying any medical terminology that may be used regarding the location of the pain, as well as discussion of the available pain relieving measures and equipment. As well as teaching the patient, it is also necessary to involve other people who may have any contact with the patient, by suggesting ways in which they can assist by providing information of the pain relieving measures which have been found to be effective.

The patient should be encouraged to take adequate rest and relaxation and there are many things which can be done to increase the patient's comfort. Such measures will be based on a knowledge of the things which help the patient to relax or sleep. Various measures might include the use of muscle relaxants and/or tranquillisers, which can enhance the effect of analgesia, if administered simultaneously. While they do not in themselves relieve pain, they are very valuable in promoting relaxation by reducing muscle tension. Sedatives may also be very useful in inducing sleep. Adequate sleep of the right type is essential and the patient must feel sufficiently rested and to have obtained benefit from his sleep. Inadequate rest means that the patient will be tense and will feel his pain more intensely. While medication for some patients may be the answer, the need for a quiet, comfortable environment must not be forgotten.

The nurse can make sure that the patient is well positioned and supported when in bed, that the bed is comfortable and the bed clothes are not heavy or restricting; she should attend to the patient's physical hygiene and see that the skin is clean and dry. In other words, basic nursing techniques are as important as adequate pain relieving drugs. The patient should be encouraged to take a nourishing diet and the maintenance of optimal nutrition is important in keeping the patient alert, mobile and interested in his surroundings. The application of heat to painful limbs often relieves pain, which in turn helps to improve mobility. Skin sensation may be impaired and care must be taken that burns do not occur. If there is respiratory distress associated with respiratory infection, the administration of Tinct. Benz. Co. or menthol inhalations can help to promote expectoration. Skilled physiotherapy can be invaluable.

The nurse should ensure that adequate analgesia is given prior to any procedure which may cause pain, e.g. change of position. Such medication should be given so that the procedure can coincide with the maximum analgesic effect. When the patient is reasonably comfortable at rest but is gravely distressed on being turned, as may be the case with bone metastases, an effective potent short-acting analgesic such as Entonox, can be used. Entonox is a mixture of 50 per cent oxygen and 50 per cent nitrous oxide, and can be self-administered via a face mask or a mouth piece by the patient. This avoids the danger of overdosage as the mask will fall away from the patient's face automatically when sufficient Entonox is inhaled. The advantages of Entonox are now being realised as a convenient and safe way of administering a quick acting, short-term analgesia.

The management of pain is complex and demands a multi-disciplinary approach. It is important for the nurse to understand the background to pain causation and pain management. It is even more important for the nurse to realise that it is her approach and sympathetic understanding of a patient's needs which is as important (in some cases, more important) as medical relief of pain. To help a patient through periods of physical pain and to see him relaxed and comfortable as the result of good treatment, can be most rewarding to the nurse.

REFERENCES

Benoliel, J. Q. and Crowley, D. M. (1974). *The Patient in Pain: New Concepts*. American Cancer Society Professional Education Publication.

McCaffery, M. (1972). *Nursing Management of the Patient with Pain*. Lippincott, New York.

Melzack, R. (1973). *The Puzzle of Pain*. Penguin Educational, London.

Sternback, R. A. (1974). *Pain: Patients, Traits and Treatment*. Academic Press, New York.

Twycross, R. G. (1975). A Symposium on Pain. *British Medical Journal*, **4**, 212.

A Symposium on Pain (1977). *Nursing Mirror*, **144**, 10.

10. Terminal Care
by MARJOLIJN KRAUSS SRN, DN(Lond.)

Terminal care means essentially the care of the living, and is the care given to a patient in the last phase of life. The fear of death is a universal one. It exists within each normal person and has persisted since the evolution of man. It is impossible to conceive what death exactly means to ourselves, even though we are able to relate it to others. Basically, we resist the idea that our life, thoughts and emotions must, with death, come to an abrupt halt. Mankind has searched for many means to relieve this fear and most religions embody some belief in the after-life, which gives some form of reassurance to our existence; that the end death brings is not a total cessation of life, but that it continues in some other form. These beliefs are often expressed in the euphemisms that the dead person has 'passed on', 'fallen asleep' or 'gone to the other side'.

Death may be discussed impartially as occurring to others, but most people are unwilling to discuss the actual process of dying. A recent (1977) 'Man Alive' television programme studied society's attitudes to death and showed that death still remains very much a taboo subject. More important it also showed that the fearful aura surrounding death is accentuated by the attitudes of the caring professions within our hospitals. In this century the structure of the family has undergone many changes. Previously, because of the caring role of the extended family, many people would have died within their own homes, but it is now estimated that 60 to 70 per cent die in institutions. This makes it essential that nurses and doctors examine their own attitudes towards death. By attempting to conceal death many hospitals fail to recognise the dignity inherent in the dying process. One member of the medical profession has stated publicly that he was afraid not of death, but of dying in an institution. This is a terrible condemnation of our hospitals and one which deserves far greater attention.

TERMINAL CARE

The fear of dying and death has been discussed in many books and articles over recent years, and one might assume that staff members in hospitals dealing so frequently with death would become specialists on the subject. Researchers like Kubler-Ross, Glaser and Strauss, have shown that whilst dying is one of the most singular events in human experience, it is often an artificially prolonged and dehumanising agony endured in an atmosphere of isolation. It seems that while medical science has freed man from ignorance, it has so far failed to provide a satisfying understanding of the meaning of life and death. The past decades have not only seen medical advances, but also a decline or change in religious attitudes. Religion played an important function and often took over when medical treatment failed, by reassuring the patient that suffering had a meaning and would be rewarded in the next life. Today there are fewer patients who hold any strong convictions in a life after death. The dying patient may thus be forced to accept the reality of his impending death without the comfort that faith previously brought.

Nurses need to examine critically their own profession in order to come to terms with the subject of dying and thereby improve their care given to the dying patient. Throughout the education of the nurse, subjects relating to terminal care and the care of their relatives remain neglected. Nurses cannot be expected to cope with these situations if inadequate guidance is given to them during training by physicians, educators and other health care professionals.

Can one, in reality, teach about terminal care? The subject only becomes a meaningful experience when dying is seen not as a failure of care, but rather as a completion of care. Too often the nurse who is told to bed bath the dying patient is the most junior member of the ward team. This is the time the patient is most likely to ask those searching questions which an inexperienced nurse dreads. Frequently, the ward sister emphasises avoidance by moving the patient, who is seldom consulted, into the corner bed of a ward or into a side room. Patients are subjected to the macabre scene of the 'death trolley' being wheeled away in the silent pretence that it is just an ordinary trolley. Can any doctor or

TERMINAL CARE

nurse really believe that death can be hidden behind screens or that such conspiracies of silence protect patients from fear? Most patients in a ward are acutely aware of those who are deteriorating and by witnessing high standards of care and attention given openly to them, they can see that nurses, as a profession, can bring a quiet form of dignity to death. This, unlike the avoidance situations described above, is essentially the completion of care.

Fear of abandonment is considered by some psychologists to be one of the basic fears of mankind. Even in adult life people are inescapably dependent upon each other for their mental health. Erich Fromm in *The Fear of Freedom* wrote, 'To feel completely alone and isolated leads to mental disintegration just as physical starvation leads to death.' The terminal patient alas, is often isolated both physically and emotionally. If dying patients are asked whether they would like to be moved, many express a fear of being isolated in a single room. They are capable of associating this with impending death, despite any other plausible reasons given to them. There are patients who would appreciate the privacy of a room and if they have been asked then at least they have been involved in the decision making. The question which ought to be raised is whether it should ever become a ward routine to move dying patients, especially if they are being kept comfortable? What are the motives? In some cases it is done to protect the other patients but often to protect the staff. Yet, does it in fact, protect anyone? If one gently questions the other patients in a ward, they are often fully aware about the reasons for moving terminal patients and as a result their own fears concerning death may be worsened. It is to be hoped that the needs of each patient will be assessed individually; wherever possible the patient and his relatives should be fully involved in the decision relating as to where he wishes to remain.

There have been a number of research projects, notably in America, which have studied the attitudes of the nurse towards dying patients. These projects have shown that many nurses are afraid of confrontation with a terminal patient and that they will avoid spending too much time with them. This fear is a very real one; nurses are often involved in a conspiracy of deception in which the truth remains hidden from the patient. In some cases this occurs because of attitudes held by doctors, but it may also happen because the relatives insist on keeping the truth from the patient. The deception continues today despite an increasing number of publications which show that it rarely succeeds in what it sets out to do; namely to protect the patient from the truth. John Hinton in his study of dying, visited patients in a general hospital throughout the course of their illness and took particular note of the comments they made about their expectation of recovery. Some were known to have fatal illnesses, others less serious conditions. His experience led him to two important conclusions. One was that regardless of what they had been told, the majority of terminal patients were aware that they were dying. The other was that the opportunity to talk about such disturbing possibilities was viewed very positively by the patients. Far from stirring up discontent on the ward by upsetting the patients, he found that most patients were glad to discuss their fears openly.

Many nurses now feel that the patient should be told the truth about his illness and in time it is to be hoped that the conflict will not be whether or not to tell a patient, but how to tell him. It is not easy for anyone to tell a patient of his fatal illness, but once this has been done, all those who are concerned in his care must take the responsibility to help him come to terms with the truth. The words in a Simon and Garfunkel song, 'a man hears what he wants to hear and disregards the rest' explains clearly the process of denial. Physicians may indeed decide to tell: the patient will decide what he accepts. The whole caring team should be prepared for such reactions and understand that whilst truth is desirable, denial mechanisms work to protect the patient from painful reality. The nurse needs to learn and understand that denial is not necessarily a negative mechanism, but often a means of coming to terms with the truth.

The concept of terminal care units has arisen because many busy medical and surgical wards are claimed to be bad places in which to die as the staff may be preoccupied with heroic efforts to save life. Amid the resuscitation equipment the terminal patient may be seen as a sad failure. It is here that attitudes play a vital part, because if the inevitable progression of a disease is accepted, any hospital ward can become a peaceful place in which to die. In such a situation, measures for the prolongation of life are considered only when there is a reasonable chance that the quality of the life that remains will justify the means to prolong it.

In terminal care the priority is symptomatic treatment, which may or may not prolong life. In the care of the patient suffering from a malignant condition, treatment involves radiotherapy, further surgery, treatment with cytotoxic drugs and hormones. The nurse's advice may be asked by the patient or relatives and for this reason it is essential that the nurse has a clear understanding of the disease process together with knowledge of both the beneficial as well as side-effects of treatments offered to the patient. There are many examples in cancer nursing; it is recognised that patients with bone metastases are liable to develop pathological fractures, hypercalcaemia, cord compression and anaemia; severe anaemia could precipitate heart failure and pulmonary oedema; cord compression could lead rapidly to paraplegia; and brain metastases could produce convulsions and personality changes. These are but a few examples of problems which may occur and if left untreated certainly diminish the quality of life. It is the responsibility of all ward sisters to alert their staff to the signs and symptoms of complications and at all times be prepared to offer explanations of treatment. Nurses may find themselves in the position where the question of the ethical use of certain forms of treatment arises; at such times the nurse needs to remember that hope is important to the patient. Hinshaw (1969), wrote '... the skilled physician's estimate of the vague factor of a tenacious hold upon life, which defies description but is none the less of considerable importance.' The patient may fear the side-effects of treatment, but he fears the abandonment of all medical treatment even more.

In a rapidly advancing technological society, the nurse has to become increasingly more alert to the scientist in the doctor. While no nurse should assume the responsibility that a doctor has to his patient, she can ensure that the patient and relatives are informed and involved in the decision making regarding further treatment. She must also acquire the courage of her convictions and be prepared to voice the patient's wishes when he feels he cannot endure any more side-effects of treatment. This is never easy and nurses need to be experienced and mature in order that they are not influenced by their emotional involvement with their patients. Any questions raised should be objective, well reasoned, and motivated only by attaining the best care possible for the patient. It is also to be hoped that the medical staff will involve the nursing staff fully and will be prepared to give clear explanations of the rationale of treatment. This will lead to true teamwork. Once treatment has been started the patient and his relatives may need a great deal of support and reassurance to persevere with it. The side-effects of most forms of treatment are usually temporary and the long-term benefits to the patient may far outweigh these unpleasant symptoms. Every effort is required to minimise unpleasant symptoms and reassure the patient that once treatment has been completed, these side-effects will disappear. The care of the terminal patient is based on the firm belief that nothing is hopeless and that when treatment has failed to halt the progress of his disease, his physical and mental comfort become the overriding priority.

In trying to help a patient through his terminal illness, doctors and nurses are taking part in a process of psychological transition which, like grief, requires time, empathy and trust. A ward in which the spiritual and psychological resources of the whole nursing and medical team enable them to accept death as a meaningful event, and in which the psychological as well as the physical needs of the patient are the central concern of everybody, can enable patients, in time, to talk about the various fears and anxieties that trouble them. In such a ward the patients soon discover that the staff want to know them as people and where actually sitting down and talking with patients is regarded as part of their work.

So far, terminal care has been discussed against a background of staff attitudes and present day conflicts; no chapter on terminal care would be complete if it did not include the general emotional responses which may be witnessed in terminal patients and their relatives. Though not all patients die from cancer, it is the disease which carries the greatest emotional impact. Few people would choose to die of cancer, since to many it means prolonged physical pain and suffering, as well as physical disability and deterioration. It may mean loss of independence and it can create social and psychological isolation if loved ones are afraid of the disease or of death. When cancer is a terminal condition, it usually leaves time for reflection of one's life – a time which can be emotionally painful when there are regrets.

Mailer in his novel, *An American Dream*, writes: 'In some, madness must come in with breath, mill through the blood and be breathed out again. In some it goes up to the mind. Some take the madness and stop it with discipline. Madness is locked beneath. It goes into tissues, is swallowed by the cells. The cells go mad. Cancer is their flag. Cancer is the growth of madness denied. In that corpse I saw, madness went down to the blood – leucocytes gorged the liver, the spleen, the enlarged heart and violet-black lungs, dug into the intestines, germinated stench.' Such descriptions cannot fail to produce some form of fear in anyone reading them. Thus any emotional response needs to be seen in terms of what the patient perceives cancer to be. The word cancer may be perceived as an invasion, tissue destruction creating 'holes' in the body or 'eating away' organs; it may mean severe pain, helplessness and death. The emotional responses run a complete cross-section from total denial of the illness on one extreme to delusional cancer phobia on the other. Each person has highly individual responses to the process of their illness, and many of these responses are based on childhood experiences with sickness and their parents' reactions to illness. When a patient is aware that something serious is wrong with him, he employs mental mechanisms that are used commonly in all areas of life. Some of these responses are denial, anger, anxiety, depression, dependency and acceptance.

Denial is the most frequently used defence mechanism and it is purposeful. It is a healthy reaction in all normal people in order to give one time to adapt and later draw on other defence mechanisms, it acts as a buffer after the shock of hearing bad news. There are several forms of denial; the patient may recognise the nature of cancer but refuses to accept anything other than an overtly optimistic view; he may recognise the existence of cancer but fails to be concerned and this may be achieved through strong religious beliefs, conscious avoidance of the subject or an apathetic approach; and thirdly, the patient may refuse to accept the situation as posing a threat to his life. Denial may be a means to avoid psychological disability or in its most extreme form, comprise a symptom of mental disorder. One has always to remain cautious in dealing with patients using this defence mechanism. It may not be advisable to counter denial, as denial for the patient may be essential if he is to maintain his emotional stability. Periods of denial are seen throughout the patient's illness. It is virtually impossible for even the most well adjusted person to remain continuously realistic about a life threatening illness. Excessive denial leading to apathetic withdrawal is a more serious and difficult problem to deal with and sometimes excessive fear may be the root cause.

Once the shock of bad news wears off and denial can no longer be maintained, it is often replaced by resentment and anger. This, once again, is a very natural human response. All of us will have reacted to serious situations with an anger which asks the universal question 'Why me?' Such response by the patient can cause distress to relatives and friends and can certainly lead to his being regarded as an 'unpopular patient'. His anger is often indiscriminate and it may be difficult to do anything to please him. Whether nurses agree with it or not, they possess certain formulated standards of what is 'expected' from patients, tending to expect them to maintain relative composure and dignity in face of illness. How many nurses, placed in the patient's position – confined and restricted to the hospital environment; undergoing prolonged and sometimes uncomfortable tests and treatment; trying to accept that time has limitations; frightened of becoming dependent on others when previously one has been independent; afraid to show fear and anxiety – would be able to remain calm and composed under such stresses?

Each patient with terminal cancer responds with anxiety and

depression. The degree with which these occur varies with each individual personality. For some, these emotions become pathological; for others they are merely an expression of stress with which the patient copes successfully. Many of the emotional problems of the patient are related to his inability to handle the intensity and duration of anxiety. The presence of anxiety may significantly enhance discomfort which is described as 'increased pain'. There is no doubt that many patients benefit from drugs or other means that alleviates their anxiety and thereby become less sensitive to discomfort or pain. Anxiety may show itself in many forms, such as nervousness, agitation, tension, aggressiveness and insomnia. It is a well known fact that the level of anxiety increases at night when there is little to distract the thoughts of the patient. At such times, a sympathetic night nurse who understands the increased anxiety and makes time to listen and reassure instead of offering more sedation, can provide help of far greater value.

Another anticipated emotional response to cancer is the depressed mood. This may be mild or transitory, often without obvious symptoms of the depressed syndrome. If it develops to a greater extent, added symptoms of guilt and self-deprecation are often seen, with pre-occupation of self and the symptoms of the illness. A negative outlook may occur and is maintained towards self, family, hospital staff and the world in general, and it becomes obvious that the activities and interests which the patient usually enjoyed are no longer pleasurable. Kubler-Ross in *On Death and Dying* defined two kinds of depression – 'When the depression is a toll to prepare for impending loss of all loved objects, in order to facilitate the state of acceptance, then encouragements and reassurance are not as meaningful. The patient should not be encouraged to look at the sunny side of things, as this would mean that he should not contemplate his impending death. It would be contra-indicated to tell him not to be sad, since all of us are tremendously sad when we lose one beloved person. The patient is in the process of losing everything and everybody he loves. If he is allowed to express his sorrow he will find real acceptance much easier and he will be grateful to those who can sit with him during this stage of depression without constantly telling him not to be sad. This type of depression is usually a silent one, in contrast to the reactive depression during which the patient requires many verbal interactions ...'.

There are other causes for depression – it is a common feature of cytotoxic chemotherapy and radiotherapy, though the exact reason is not known. It is also common in those who face long and extensive surgery and in those patients who are old and lonely, with few visitors during their stay in hospital. In all cases, nurses are the observers of depression and should attempt to elicit the cause before making sweeping assumptions that it is solely due to the malignant process. The nurse may benefit from contact and discussion with the relatives and once the cause is elicited, the relatives should always be included in the attempts made to cope with this problem.

Another response frequently encountered in hospital is an exaggeration of the human dependency need. Most people during the process of normal development spend an extended period of time in dependency relationships within the family. Initially in infancy this is a biological dependency that is extended as social and economic dependency into young adulthood. Behavioural responses and anticipations are therefore built into any life situation which involves dependency needs and feelings and the problem of dependency versus independence is a life long issue. When a situation of stress develops, one often resorts to some form of dependency. Some people cope with a remarkable degree of stoicism; some feel the need to share but are unable to ask for help, some immediately resort to the desire for complete care. The need to share and the need to depend upon someone else in times of stress is completely natural as no man is 'an island unto themselves' (Donne). Yet in hospitals dependency is a two-edged sword; it may help the patient psychologically or prevent him from ever coming to terms with his life situation. The sensitive nurse will detect imminent psychological invalidism and seek assistance to prevent the development of such negative attitudes. Nurses need to be careful not to deprive a terminal patient of his need for independence and decision making.

There usually comes a stage when all or some of the previous emotional responses have run their course and the patient comes to terms with his condition. The degree of acceptance often largely depends on the age, personality, social circumstances and general condition of the patient. He may have denied or fought against the reality of his disease; he may have searched all the channels which offered him some hope; he will have been depressed and anxious. Slowly, his mind will have begun to accept the inevitable outcome. The patient may at this stage be weak and exhausted and at such times the mind cannot cope with further stress and thus acceptance is not always a state of peace – it may simply be a state of mind which says 'I've had enough'. During such periods, his interests in his surroundings, friends and family may actually decline. What are the patient's thoughts at this time? None can tell, but physical and emotional exhaustion does cause the thought processes to become dulled and diminished. It can be a trying time for the relatives and nurses as acceptance is often regarded as 'giving up'. However disturbing it may be to an onlooker, this acceptance should be regarded as natural in a patient for whom no further curative treatment is available. It is difficult to refrain from attempting to remain encouraging and trying to instil further hope to the patient. He simply needs the quiet presence of his loved ones and their acceptance of his resignation. Relatives also need support at this time. They may attempt to awaken the patient's interests and can become upset when he fails to respond, and it is at this time that they need to begin to prepare themselves for the grief reaction which will follow his death.

A young patient does not easily accept his terminal condition; some never accept it and never give up hope. At times their bitter struggle to remain alive can be traumatic to all who witness it. Many doctors and nurses find it difficult to deal with this situation; the patient is often in the same age group as those caring for him, with the result that they may over-identify with his rejection of reality. Society tends to praise those who never give up fighting for their life, but it rarely considers the mental anguish this expectation can cause. The care of these patients requires all the resources a team effort can provide, and it should never be left as the responsibility of one person alone. Senior medical and nursing staff should be very alert to the effects such situations may have on the younger and less mature members of their staff and be willing to counsel and give guidance.

Patients who come from broken homes or life situations which have been filled with friction and a lack of love need special consideration. Every person needs love and affection, and this need does not diminish; it may become stronger at this time. The patient may have reviewed his past life and seen where he failed in love, or where others have failed him. Some patients may be ignored or rejected at this stage, with few visitors to give them the reassurance they need, and in these situations, it is the nursing staff who have to fulfil the needs to some degree. Often it is the fear of becoming too involved emotionally which prevents one from doing this; this failure then becomes a reflection of emotional immaturity. One patient, a woman aged 45, who was dying from breast cancer, wrote in her diary: 'Often, when seriously ill, we are subject to doubts, fears and anxiety and feel the intense desire to talk to someone who understands and can give a little hope, strength and courage. At this time more than any other time in life, do we confront our real and true self.'

The care of the relatives is an integral part of terminal care and the manner in which we may impart such care may later determine how they are able to cope with their grief reactions. The relatives bear the burden of the illness that afflicts their loved ones. For them life must go on. They are expected to support, encourage and give hope and yet in the case of an incurable patient, may have to face a long period in which to prepare themselves for the final loss of their relative. Relatives may at times stand in awe of the medical profession and feel uncomfortable in the hospital environment. This may be accentuated when information which is incomprehensible is given to them, which leaves them bewildered and confused. There is a temptation amongst the caring professions to cloak their own inadequacies in a jargon of medical expressions. Every attempt should be made to explain details in understandable terms and nurses should be prepared to repeat this on numerous occasions. The whole ward team should know what has been said to relatives, and so prevent them being given conflicting information.

Relatives will often show similar psychological responses as described earlier in relation to the patient. Once they are informed about the poor prognosis, they are placed in a stress situation and their first reaction may be complete disbelief. Either they do not believe that the doctor has made the correct diagnosis or if they accept the diagnosis, then they refuse to believe that their loved one is as ill as they are told. After such news has been imparted, each person comes to terms with it in their own way, though some will try to remain unrealistically optimistic long after the doctors have ceased active treatment. To understand why some relatives do this, the nurse must look at the events which frequently lead up to this. In the normal course of events the consultant becomes aware of the true situation after tests, examinations or operation. He then breaks the news to the relatives, whom he has probably never met before. Often this news is not given to the patient, which may lead him to believe that there is no cause for alarm. The reason behind this is the assumption that bad news would depress him and that if he is going to die it is kinder to protect him from the truth. The relatives, however, must be told and they often do their utmost to keep the truth from the patient. It is rarely appreciated how difficult this task is.

The whole family is under stress and such situations disrupt the customary modes of behaviour of the people concerned. Just how they react to stress depends on many factors – the type of stressful situation; the individual's defence mechanisms; his perception of the situation and his capacity to tolerate anxiety. It is hardly surprising that the behavioural responses vary widely. Anger is not an uncommon emotion and is often directed against the caring professions. While some of the anger may be irrational it can well be understood that relatives need to blame someone or something for their impending loss. Often there is a feeling that if the person responsible could be found, the situation may improve. It is at such times that nurses have to learn to cope with critical and sometimes abusive behaviour, but it is important to allow the relatives to openly express their feelings and not to engage in a conflict. Anger may isolate the relatives from the medical and nursing staff at the time when their support is most needed.

Since the length of the terminal stage is never predictable, the family may have to cope with this stressful situation for weeks or even many months. In order to provide good care, the family members should not be left to feel helpless and they must know that they will be supported. There are families who become exhausted long before the ordeal is over, not because of physical fatigue, but from the prolonged period during which individual family members do not have the means of meeting their own personal needs. When a family reaches this state, the desire to 'get it over with' often generates feelings of resentment towards the dying person, as well as guilt for feeling that way. These feelings add to the burdens of the grief process and can be reduced by the sympathetic nurse, who is aware that her care of the patient also includes the family.

There is a growing awareness of the importance of terminal care and the need for more guidance and support to all who are involved, as indicated in two recent reports. The British Medical Association report on *Care of the Elderly* (July 1976) stated that 'little attention is paid to the care of the dying in the training of doctors and nurses, social workers and all who have a professional role to play need more training in this special skill . . . allied to this need for training in the care of the dying is the need for fuller appreciation of the problems of the bereaved . . . involving relatives in the terminal care process is perhaps the most important factor in ensuring that, when death finally comes to a patient, they will be able to accept this in a realistic and less troubled way, and be spared the abnormal bereavement reactions which can lead to prolonged emotional ill health.' The report of the *Evidence to the Royal Commission on the National Health Service* by the Royal College of Nursing (March 1977) made a similar observation: 'The health and social services need to make better provisions for terminal care which has been relatively neglected because it is considered of less importance than acute medicine. But since Western culture deems that people should be born and die in institutions, it should ensure that the peace and dignity are no less than would be experienced at home and the patients and their relatives are supported with understanding and sympathy to the last.'

This chapter has concentrated on the care of terminal patients in hospital; this does not ignore the fact that the most suitable place for a patient to die would be his own home. Terminal care at home is demanding for both the doctor, community nurse and relatives and its success depends largely on a co-ordinated effort by the whole primary health care team. If this can be attained, it must surely be the most rewarding aspect of primary care.

In the effort to improve terminal care, the nurse should beware of making the care of the dying a speciality and be tempted to follow too many formulated theories. People will face death in much the same way as they face life. The danger of too many theories is that it may be used as a defence instead of a means to understanding and growth. This danger was so clearly reflected in the poetry of a young man dying of leukaemia. Ted Rosenthal in his *How Could I not Be Amongst You* wrote 'All those people who say that you are predictable and that you will die in the same way that everyone else dies, they are right. I resented that at first. I resented them saying "Oh you are at the two week stage. You're feeling, doing this. You're free. You're at the angry stage. I understand that. You're depressed. You're lost. Three and one half weeks after you find this out you always feel lost". Well they're right. It works that way with me. I am following patterns. I am following the guidelines for dying of terminal cancer patients down to the letter. They all told me how this would be, how I would be reacting. It's fiendish. No matter what I say, they say "Hm. That's what we thought you'd say". Especially the nurses – and the doctors too. All of them.'

Words from the report of the British Medical Association make an apt conclusion: 'Policies regarding admission to hospital of those suffering from terminal illness should be interpreted as liberally as possible, and prompt action taken when the need is established. Old people should not be left to die alone or in unrelieved pain, or as victims of squalor, incontinence or neglect.

Death may be inevitable, but it should not be without dignity and a lack of a home in which to die may, in many cases, leave no alternative to hospital care.'

REFERENCES

Glaser, B. G. and Strauss, A. L. (1964). The Social Loss of Dying Patients. *American Journal of Nursing*, **64**, 6.

Glaser, B. G. and Strauss, A. L. (1966). *Awareness of Dying. A Sociological Study of Attitudes toward the Patient Dying in Hospital*. Weidenfeld and Nicolson, London.

Hinshaw, H. C. (1969). *Diseases of the Chest*. W. B. Saunders and Co., Philadelphia.

Hinton, J. (1963). The Physical and Mental Distress of the Dying. *Quarterly Journal of Medicine*, **32**, 1.

Hinton, J. (1967). *Dying*. Penguin Books, London.

Kubler-Ross, E. (1970). *On Death and Dying*. Tavistock Publications, London.

Rosenthal, T. (1973). *How Could I Not Be Amongst You?* George Braziller Inc., New York.

Care of the Elderly (1976). Report of the British Medical Association.

Evidence to the Royal Commission on the National Health Service. Royal College of Nursing (1977). Whitefriars Press.

BIBLIOGRAPHY

Capra, L. G. (1972). *The Care of the Cancer Patient*. William Heinemann Medical Books Ltd., London.

Lamerton, R. (1973). *Care of the Dying*. Priory Press.

Parkes, C. Murray (1975). *Bereavement*. Pelican Books, London.

Peterson, B. H. and Kellog, C. J. (1976). *Current Practice in Oncological Nursing*. Volume 1. C. V. Mosby and Co., St Louis.

Saunders, C. (1976). *Care of the Dying*. (2nd Ed.). Reprint from *Nursing Times*, Macmillan Press.

Index

actinomycin D, 54, 102, 104
adrenalectomy, 62, 65
adrenal insufficiency, 69
Adriamycin, 54, 93, 102, 104, 134
alopecia, 45, 145
anaemia, 42, 43, 68, 175
androgens, 62, 64
  side-effects of, 62
anti-tumour drugs – *see* chemotherapy
L-asparaginase, 54, 104

BCG, 135, 141
bleomycin, 55, 76, 86, 106
blood count, 39
blood pressure, 70
bone marrow:
  biopsy, 40
  depression, 42
  transplant, 116, 122, 125, 130
bowel care, 45, 47, 67
breast cancer, 21, 30, 32
  chemotherapy for, 35
  influence of hormones on, 60–4
  in men, 63
bronchus, oat cell carcinoma of, 21
  chemotherapy for, 31, 36
busulphan, 51

cell, 22
  cycle, 22, 28
  kinetics, 22–4, 27, 30
cell separator, 125, 130–45
  drug overdose, treatment by, 145
  granulocyte transfusions, 142
  method of use of, 135
  nursing care of patient on, 138–41
  plasma exchange, 144
  Rhesus antibody collection, by, 145
chemotherapy:
  adjuvant, 24, 29–31, 35
  administration of, 40, 124
  arterial infusion, 41

bladder cancer, for, 37
breast cancer, for, 35
childhood cancers, for, 35
combination, 28, 34, 37
  empirical rules for, 29
combined with radiotherapy and surgery, 41
continuous single agent low dose, 26, 40
cyclical, 27
drug kinetics, 24
high dose intermittent, 41
high dose intermittent combination, 27, 41
intravenous infusion, 42
investigations before, 39
leukaemia, for, 38, 134
methods of testing new drugs for, 25
neutropenia following, 113
regional perfusion, 41
selectivity, 22
side-effects of, 42–58
tumour response to, 32
types of drugs used in, 49–58
chicken pox, 114, 148
childhood cancers, 21, 29, 35, 146–58
  anti-tumour drug care in, 154
  death from, 155
  infection in, 114, 148
  nurse's role, in, 146–8
  pain control in, 154
  play therapist, value of, in, 150
  radiotherapy in, 152–4
  role of parents in, 146, 151, 154–7
chlorambucil, 51, 67
chordotomy, 166, 168
classification of anti-tumour agents, 49-58
colonic cancer; chemotherapy for, 31
communications:
  nurse/doctor, 38, 68, 69, 72, 103, 175

INDEX

communications: – *contd.*
  nurse/patient, 42, 43, 62, 69, 72, 93, 103, 142, 168, 175
  patient/doctor, 62, 142
cortisone, 60
Cushing's syndrome, 69–70
cyclophosphamide, 28, 36, 51, 106
cystitis, 47
cytosine arabinoside, 49, 106, 134
cytotoxic drugs – *see* chemotherapy

dying, care of the, 155–7, 171–86
  acceptance of, 181
  fear of, 171
  nurse's role in, 171
  reactions to, 177–81
devices for intravenous therapy:
  cannulae, 77, 80
  catheters, 77, 80, 82
  obturators and stoppers, 78
  winged infusion set, 77, 79
diarrhoea, 45, 152
diet, 45, 148, 169
DNA, 22
drug research, 25
D-TIC, 89, 101, 102, 106
Durabolin, 62

electrocardiogram, 40, 48
electrolyte balance, 45, 75, 161
endocrine therapy, 35, 60–72
  side-effects of, 62, 69–72
Entonox, 95, 170
ependymoma, 30
epilation – *see* alopecia
Ewing's tumour, 29, 30
extravasation, 100, 102

fluid balance, 45, 152, 161
5-fluorouracil, 31, 49, 108
fractional cell kill principle, 23, 27

gastro-intestinal tract, 44, 71
gonads, 28, 47
growth hormone, 60

hepatitis, 115
herpes virus, 114, 117
Hodgkin's disease, 28, 31, 34

hormone therapy – *see* endocrine therapy
hydroxurea, 58, 84
hypercalcaemia, 67
  treatment of, 68
hypophysectomy, 63

IBM Cell Separator, 125 *see also* cell separator
immunotherapy, 135, 138, 141
immunological response, 113
infection:
  control of, 113–21
  detection of, 118
  epidemiology of, 117
  opportunistic, 114
    bacterial, 114
    fungal, 115
    parasitic, 116
    viral, 114
  prevention of, 118
  protecting the patient from, 116
  sources of hospital, 120
  treatment of generalised, 117
intravenous therapy, 73–112, 118
  administration sets for, 84
  cannulae for, 77, 78, 80
  care of the patient undergoing, 98–104
  catheters for, 77, 80
  choice of device for, 77
  containers for, 85–7
  devices for, 79–85
  drug administration by, 74, 75, 76, 89
  giving sets for, 83
  hazards of, 83, 101
  indications for, 73
  management of, 96
  nurse's role in implementing, 76
  parenteral feeding by, 74
  preparation of patient for, 93
  recording, 91
  solutions, 87
    DHSS policy for addition of drugs to, 89
    reactions of drugs to, 87
  venepuncture, 73, 77, 121

INDEX

investigations, prior to chemotherapy, 39
  specific:
    EDTA, 40
    GPT, 40
isolation of patient, 116, 121, 122–33
isolator tent, 133

kidney, adenocarcinoma of, 66

'leaching', 83, 86, 100
leucopenia, 42
leukaemia, 26, 28, 67, 122, 125
  acute lymphoblastic, 33, 67, 115, 154
  acute myeloblastic, 34
  acute myeloid, 125, 134
  meningopathy, 33
Leukopak, 143
lung cancer – *see* bronchus
lymphoma, 26, 34

Masteril, 62
measles, 115, 148
medulloblastoma, 30
melanoma malignant, 37
melphalan, 52, 108
6-mercaptopurine, 50
metastases, 29, 30, 175
  bone, 65, 67
  breast cancer, from, 35
  lung cancer, from, 36
methotrexate, 50, 76, 86, 98, 108
mithramycin, 56, 68
Mitomycin-C, 56, 108
mouth, care of, 44

nausea, 44, 47, 66, 140, 152
nephrotoxicity, 46
nervous system, 47
neuroblastoma, 31, 36
neurotoxicity, 28, 48
neutropenia, 113, 116, 125, 142, 149
Nitrogen mustard (mustine), 29, 36, 52, 88, 93, 108
nurse:
  attitude to cancer of, 14, 103
  role of the, 11, 76, 120, 142, 146, 168–70, 183–5
  training, 13, 172

nursing observations, 42–8, 91, 103, 140, 163, 168

oestrogen, 60, 63, 65, 67
oncology, 13
  medical, 19
oophorectomy, 61
orchidectomy, 63, 64
osteoporosis, 67
ovarian tumour, 26

pain, 154, 159–70, 179
  assessment, 163
  definition of, 159
  fear of, 167
  measurement of, 164
  methods of control and relief of, 162, 165–70
  nature of, 160–2
  reaction to, 159
pain scale gauge, 165
parenteral feeding, 74–5
pathogen free environment, 43, 116, 122–3, 135
  admission to, 129
  care of patients in, 130
  cell separator in, 125
  cooking in, 128
  medical care of patients in, 129
  preparation of patient for a, 126
  sterilisation of equipment, 126–8
petechiae, 43
pituitary gland, 61, 63
platinum, 54, 98, 108
Platt Committee, 146
prednisone, 67, 68
pressure areas, 46, 72
procarbazine, 58
progesterone, 60, 64, 65–6, 67
prolactin, 61
prostatic cancer, hormone influence on, 64
pulmonary system, 48

remission of disease, 26, 27, 33, 34, 64, 135
renal cancer, 66
reverse barrier nursing – *see* pathogen free environment

rhabdomyosarcoma, 29, 36
rhizotomy, 166
RNA, 22
Rubidomycin, 55, 106

septicaemia, 43, 131
skin, care of, 46, 62
sleep, 169
steroids, side-effects of, 69, 72
survival rates, 30, 33, 36, 65

tamoxifen, 63
team liaison, 38, 73, 75, 175–6, 181–2
terminal care, 171–86
  concept of special units for, 174
  home, 185
  symptomatic treatment in, 175
testicular teratoma, 21, 30, 37
thiotepa, 52
thrombocytopenia, 43, 130
thyroid cancer, 66

tumours, animal, 25
  chemosensitivity of, 31–3
  index substances, 31

ultraviolet light, 122, 128
urinary system, 46
uterine cancer, 65

vaccinations, 149
venepuncture, 73, 77, 121
vinblastine, 57, 110
vinca alkaloids, 47, 102
vincristine, 28, 57, 110
vomiting, 44, 47

Wilms' tumour, 29, 30

xenografts, 25

yttrium implant, 63